"When I first met Dr. Eaker, I was impressed by his kind demeanor and humble approach. As I got to k   tine
love for people and a gentle spiri   and
desire to help these women in n   vho
is waiting for this valuable infor

—Florence i   ̌

Personality Plus and *Silver Boxes*

"I would never have guessed that a man could truly understand what a woman goes through when traveling life's hormonal highway, but Dr. Eaker has proved me wrong! A true blessing from God, Dr. Ron Eaker is a doctor, counselor, teacher, and friend. Not only do I recommend this book to every woman, but also to every man that desires to understand this hormonal roller coaster women experience."

—*Kathleen Jackson*, Publisher of *The Godly Business Woman* Magazine

"Ron Eaker has given us a road map to healthier, happier living. Wise and witty, frank and faithful, Ron weaves medicine and religion together, as God surely intended them to be. Then, step by step, he invites the reader to move in the right direction. I recommend his book to any woman who is dealing with menopause, and to the man who loves her!"

—*Dr. David Jones*, Pastor

"When hormonal issues hit us, our usually cheerful countenance becomes a fearful confusion. We feel more hostile than holy; ashamed of our actions, uncomfortable with our bodies, and too embarrassed to ask for help. In one comprehensive guide, Dr. Eaker provides women of all ages hope for their female concerns."

—*Marita Littauer*, President, CLASServices Inc.

"I found this book to be truly informative, spiritual, and humorous. . . . Dr. Eaker uses the Bible to show us that God does have a plan in menopause . . . [Dr. Eaker] is quick to point out that WE control our way of thinking. . . . He shows us some very realistic goals, and how to best achieve them, by taking them one at a time! Dr. Eaker is quick to offer advice on methods for dealing with PMS and menopause . . . [including] hormonal therapy . . .

herbs, diet, . . . [and] our spiritual well being. He is a wealth of information on other sources to gather the information we seek: the Bible, other publications, and of course, the Internet. . . . Thank you, Dr. Eaker, for helping me to see the things that were just beyond my view, and teaching me what I need to do to help myself through changes . . . [toward] the glory that can be found in menopause!"

—*Darci Warner*, TheParentClub.com

"This book deals with much more than hormones; though it thoroughly covers those topics. It is an inspirational book for choosing a healthy lifestyle. It is intertwined with Scripture, stories, and a good dose of humor. I hope this book will be as meaningful to you as it has been for me."

—*Tamsen Delong*, Nurse

"I really was blessed, encouraged, and ministered to by your writings. I have recommended it to my pastor's wife and several of my friends who are struggling with the same issues as I."

—*T. Smith*, Fort Wayne, Indiana

"Dr. Eaker is amazingly intuitive, funny, and compassionate. I can't begin to tell you the difference this book made in my life. Highly recommended read for all of my friends."

—*Laurel Banks*, Amazon.com reviewer

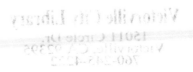

A WOMAN'S GUIDE TO
HORMONE HEALTH

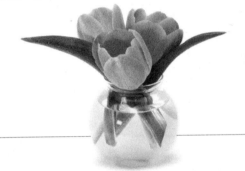

J. Ron Eaker, MD

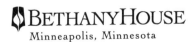
BETHANYHOUSE
Minneapolis, Minnesota

Published by Bethany House Publishers
11400 Hampshire Avenue South
Bloomington, Minnesota 55438

Bethany House Publishers is a division of
Baker Publishing Group, Grand Rapids, Michigan.

Printed in the United States of America

In keeping with biblical principles of creation stewardship, Baker Publishing Group advocates the responsible use of our natural resources. As a member of the Green Press Initiative, our company uses recycled paper when possible. The text paper of this book is comprised of 30% post-consumer waste.

green press INITIATIVE

Library of Congress Cataloging-in-Publication Data

Eaker, J. Ron.
    A woman's guide to hormone health : the Creator's way for managing menopause / J. Ron Eaker.
        p. cm.
    Summary: "Easy-to-understand, straightforward information about what's happening to women's bodies as they near and reach menopause that dispels myths about change of life, provides tips for a healthy lifestyle, and discusses treatment options"—Provided by publisher.
    Includes bibliographical references.
    ISBN 978-0-7642-0414-2 (pbk. : alk. paper)   1. Menopause—Popular works.
2. Menopause—Religious aspects—Christianity.   3. Middle-aged women—Health and hygiene—Popular works.   I.   Title.
    RG186.E256   2008
    618.1/75—dc22

                                                                                    2007034450

To God, who is the Great Healer, and to his glory.

To the women in my life who taught me love, respect, and faith: Dot Bouldin (Mom), my wife, Susan, and our daughters, Katie and Caroline. This book would not have been written if it weren't for their encouragement, teaching, compassion, tolerance, and unending love.

To my in-laws, Dr. and Mrs. William C. Shirley, who not only share their most precious possession, their beautiful daughter, but who also continue to inspire me as a physician. Bill is a man truly in love with the wonder of medicine.

And finally, to my patients: May they read, take action, and learn to celebrate life and all God has provided.

J. RON EAKER, MD is a board-certified obstetrician and gynecologist with 20 years' experience in medical practice. Listed in *America's Best Doctors*, he is a member of numerous professional societies and the author of *Fat-Proof Your Family*. He has appeared on several TV and radio shows, including *Life Today with James Robison*, Moody Radio, and *Janet Parshall's America*. Ron and his wife, Susan, have two daughters and live in Augusta, Georgia.

ACKNOWLEDGMENTS

The most common question I was asked after my first book, *Fat-Proof Your Family*, was published was "When are you going to write another book?" My stock answer was "When I become so passionate about something that I can't sleep at night!" I soon realized that as an obstetrician, not sleeping at night is not a good gauge of anything other than the inconsiderate nature of babies and their arrival times.

Writing another book is no small feat; it's one that requires, at a minimum, a profound sense of need. I am convinced that God often speaks to us in our perceptions of how we can contribute. At this stage of my life I have never felt the call to mission work, never sensed a need to go to seminary, never been asked (and never will be) to join a choir, but I do feel a profound directive to help women live lives of health and happiness. Some of you may find this odd—a man desiring to pursue this quest—yet, without a great deal of psychoanalysis, I can only say that all my life experience and training has brought me to this charge.

I felt this calling was partially fulfilled with *Fat-Proof Your Family*. The enthusiastic response to this work only validated that what I was saying resonated with people. But the work is not done. *A Woman's Guide to Hormone Health* was born out of a need in my own practice. More women are entering menopause today than in any other time in history. They demand scientifically valid choices in the context of their worldview. This book provides those choices.

Every project has its champions. This project is no exception. Without these champions, this book would still be just a wish, relegated to the "what if" file of my brain. It is a true joy to express my thanks to these individuals.

Bill Jensen, my agent, and more important, my friend, is a champion and a dream maker. Without his encouragement, this book would not have found the intended audience. Kyle Duncan is a visionary in the book industry. He and his colleagues at Bethany House saw a need and had the foresight to take a risk, and for that I will always be grateful. Deb Strubel was instrumental in some of the early edits of the manuscript. Ellen Chalifoux did the final edit and made the book infinitely more readable.

Dr. G. Pat Williams, my mentor and partner in my medical practice for fifteen years, taught me more about medicine and people than anyone else. He was taken from us prematurely, but my life and the lives of his family and patients are all the richer because of his legacy. Dr. David Jones is a learned and gifted minister and was instrumental in my spiritual education. I continue to be blessed by his guidance, teaching, and friendship. I am grateful to the thousands of patients who have taught me the importance of listening and caring, and that wellness is much more than simply being disease free.

Lastly, I am eternally blessed and thankful for a wonderful wife and two amazing daughters. They inspire me, challenge me, support me, and love me. I simply cannot ask for more.

CONTENTS

INTRODUCTION

A FRESH APPROACH

Menopause is not a disease. Let me repeat, menopause is *not* a disease. It is a normal, natural, God-designed phase of life. I consider myself an optimist, and my approach to menopause is one of expansive idealism. For those of you who are experiencing significant symptoms, realizing that menopause isn't a terminal illness can be liberating! The concept of menopause as the ultimate and inevitable bad aging experience is so pervasive in this culture that it must be challenged, deflated, pummeled, and exploded from the outset. You don't have to be captive in a hormonal prison cell. Even if you feel that you are floundering in the hormonal abyss, there is hope! This is the theme of this book. God did not design you to self-destruct at fifty! If you remember little else from this book, please remember this: With knowledge comes choices, with choices comes hope, and with hope comes joy. John Maxwell said, "When there is hope in the future, there is power in the present."

BASIC PRINCIPLES OF THIS BOOK

Midlife and menopause *are* many things. You may think of them as anything from a bump in the road of life to a dead-end street. Because this book is designed for Christian women (and my mother will read it), I won't use some of the more colorful descriptions of menopause that have been volunteered over the years. Confusing, challenging, exciting, disappointing, illuminating, frustrating, and promising all correctly describe menopause. This smorgasbord of feelings, thoughts, and beliefs may define your midlife experience also.

Menopause is a normal, natural transition that is individually experienced. There are some universal similarities, but because of your unique physiology and life experiences, this time in your life is unpredictable. What your mother experienced or what Mable next door felt has little or no impact on your menopause. It doesn't follow any rule book. There is no rule book for menopause—but there is a guidebook. The Bible, God's revelational gift and our owner's manual, embodies all the wisdom and encouragement you need to celebrate menopause. Granted, the word *menopause* doesn't appear in Scripture, but the principles lived and taught by men and women of the Bible can be applied to your life starting today. The Bible lays the foundation for a house of stone to weather any midlife storms. You may experience menopause as a hurricane of hormones, but if your foundation is solid, the high tide of midlife troubles can be weathered. If you have a strong foundation of faith, education, positive attitude, and commitment, you can make midlife a time of resurgence.

God has designed a plan for this time in your life. The wisdom and guidance that can be gleaned from both the Old Testament and the New Testament can be applied daily to *your* life. Tom Minnery, vice-president of public policy for Focus on the Family, writes, "[When] I was younger, I tended to believe that certain principles were true because they were in the Bible. But year by year, as I have read much of the social research, I have come to look at this a new way—that certain principles are in the Bible because they are true. They are true and helpful for all people, regardless of whether they accept or reject the Bible's central claim."[1] These enduring biblical principles provide safe paths to walk in your search for contentment in the midst of transition.

Medically speaking, I am a "recovering traditionalist." The traditional, old-school approach to menopause—which means drugs and, if that didn't work, more drugs—has been propagated since the appearance of synthetic hormones in the 1940s. This philosophy is not only very narrow but also possibly dangerous. The drug companies want you to view menopause as a disease, since we all know that diseases demand treatment. If menopause is viewed as something to be cured, there is money to be made. The truth about this transition is not to be found in textbooks or the halls of academia but by extrapolating the experiences of millions of women.

> Menopause is defined as the cessation of menstruation for 12 consecutive months. This marks the end of a woman's reproductive years. Menopause occurs naturally around age 51.2, when the ovaries stop producing estrogen, or surgically at any age when the ovaries are removed.

The doctor's exam room is a classroom. Patients become instructors, teaching what only they can impart: their life experience. Those of you in menopause understand that the old-school approach to dealing with midlife symptoms is occasionally successful. Many women have been helped by the likes of Premarin and Provera; however, many are not satisfied—and shouldn't be—with those drugs as the only options. In fact, some have discovered that their side effects are worse than what they intend to treat!

One menopausal woman put it well: "Physicians have a duty to give a woman the best care they can provide. However, each person is ultimately responsible for his or her own health. We, the patients, need help, guidance, and a listening ear." This book provides that help and guidance. But don't forget the other point she made. Your health is *your* responsibility.

UNMET NEEDS

The hormone world was rocked a few years back when studies were reported showing that only 17 percent of women eligible to take hormones in the United States were actually taking some type of hormone replacement. Understand that this meant 83 percent of menopausal women were not on hormones. This came as a big surprise to those who just assumed everyone did it! Even more enlightening was a study that indicated that up to 80 percent of women who start on hormones stop them after two years![2] From data like this, it is not hard to understand that something is amiss in hormone heaven. I strongly suspect those numbers are even lower today, as hundreds of thousands of women stopped their hormones in the last few years due to media reports of potential side effects. The result is that needs are not being met. Many are not treating menopausal symptoms (and are hot-flashing like a nuclear reactor gone berserk!) because they are not aware of their options.

Currently in the U.S. there are an estimated 41.75 million women over the age of 50. The World Health Organization estimates that by the year 2025, 1.1 billion women would be age 50 or over. [3]

Are hormones essential to post-menopausal health? Are there alternative therapies available as viable options? These questions are not sufficiently answered by traditional medical training. Medical research necessarily focuses on the physical world: diseases and afflictions of the body. What it often neglects is the impact of our thoughts and beliefs. Certainly, few medical schools embrace the idea of divine intervention. This leads to a completely secular approach to healing, one I feel is incomplete. Indeed, if you ask the wrong questions and look in the wrong places, you will often get wrong answers. God gave us an owner's manual, and it makes sense to study, learn, and apply its teachings. What we need is a resource that combines solid medical practices and a foundational belief in God's Word, and not surprisingly, these two sources are completely compatible.

BIBLICAL GUIDANCE

The ultimate guide for how to both traverse life and achieve salvation is the Bible. It is the owner's manual that we can apply from birth to the grave. Abraham Lincoln said, "This great book [the Bible] is the best gift God has given to man. But for it, we could not know right from wrong." This makes sense, yet we persistently and selectively apply its wisdom to only parts of our lives; however, a Christian worldview demands a broader application. Many aspects of our existence are addressed by Scripture. Sometimes we are loathe to translate this understanding to our daily lives. For example, for me, and maybe some of you, it is easy to compartmentalize my spiritual life from my work, but this soon becomes restrictive and hypocritical. Our health is no exception. If the words and teachings in Scripture are a template upon which to pattern our lives, then why can't these same instructions apply to women struggling with physical and emotional issues of midlife? The obvious answer is that they most certainly can and should.

Those of you who are fighting with change-of-life issues may have already obtained and applied a great deal of knowledge about traditional and alternative approaches to menopause symptoms. (And then again, you may not have—that may be why you bought this book!) Yet you may still be struggling to achieve an internal peace. What you are missing is the third component of the healing triad: a peace and comfort in your spirit. What can help you experience real joy and peace during this transition, in addition to physical relief, is the guidance and assurance of Scripture.

Dr. S. I. McMillen wrote in his fascinating book *None of These Diseases*, "Obedience to Biblical precepts is still one of the most effective ways to prevent many of the afflictions of mankind."[4]

There is a profound misperception that science and the Bible are not compatible. The reality is that the two are complementary. The 1972 General Conference of the United Methodist Church issued a statement that said, "All truth has its source in the God of truth so that our efforts to discern the connections between faith and science, grace and nature, are useful endeavors in developing credible and communicable doctrine."[5]

The prime assumption is that God is the author of creation. Science and all that it encompasses is part of the natural universe; therefore, science is of God. Science discovers the thoughts and actions of God . . . after the fact. *Time* magazine for March 5, 1990, carried an article by Michael D. Lemonick concerning new evidence about the fall of Jericho. Lemonick said, "In matters of faith, science can never provide the ultimate answers."[6] *Faith and fact* will provide you with an unbeatable combination.

Wellness, healing, and Christian theology are so intertwined that there should be a wealth of resources available with specific biblical insights for dealing with the physical and emotional changes of menopause. There simply is not. There are a multitude of books, tapes, and videos on menopause and volumes on complementary approaches, yet these often take a New Age tangent or are limited in their scope. Thus this book grew out of a need for a reference to guide those who want a biblically based, scientifically correct, practically applied guide to menopause. This book was conceived through much prayer, and the labor was intense, yet, just as in childbirth, the result was rewarding.

> The New International Version of the Bible mentions the words *health* or *healing* 57 times.

A COMBINED APPROACH

This book's goal is to examine both traditional and nontraditional (alternative) ways of approaching menopause. Information on herbs, complementary teachings, prayer, diet, and exercise dominate this approach. But I also know that, for some, conventional approaches to this transition (especially when it comes to symptom treatment) are useful and successful. Traditional medicine, as applied to menopause, is just as spiritually sound as any other scientific endeavor. This book is about choice and responsibility, both of which are sound biblical principles. God has provided many paths to a joyous life; you must choose your path. This book is about giving you the options, detailing the consequences, and prodding you to action.

The major problem in meshing traditional and complementary approaches to health is a mistaken perception of mutual exclusivity. This is a sad and limiting assumption because it blocks many from understanding the options God has provided. These apparently diverse approaches, traditional and alternative, actually are intertwined. It is unreasonable to think that God ordains only natural approaches and shuns more traditional methods.

Choice and personal responsibility are keys to unlock a joyous menopause, and this book helps you choose the right key for your lock. Some misinformed individuals feel that if you approach menopausal symptoms with only traditional solutions (i.e., hormones), you are taking the easy way out or polluting your body. Other just as confused folks believe that those who shun conventional medicines in favor of herbs and home remedies are tree huggers. These characterizations reflect more about the accusers than the accused. There are just as many closed-minded naturalists as closed-minded traditionalists. The secret is balance, and both approaches can be of God. Your goal is to find what works for you.

THEMES

The themes for this book are multiple and simple. First, menopause is a normal change, not a disease state. Second, God has a plan to help you to truly celebrate this and any change. Third, there are choices that you need to make. Fourth, you must take action. This is an opportunity to live with passion and fulfill your mission, a mission that is not completed until the Lord decides it is time for you to come home. There once was a famous preacher who was asked whether he thought his purpose in life had already been achieved. He replied, "If I am still breathing, it hasn't been!"

> According to a nationwide government survey, 36% of U.S. adults aged 18 years and over use some form of complementary or alternative medicine. The most common alternative therapy was prayer.[7]

This is a time to take stock of the past and choose your path for the future. The choice is yours. It is a choice that is difficult, if not impossible, to make wisely without sound information and guidance. In medicine and surgery we have a ritual called informed consent. It is a process whereby a patient contemplating a surgical procedure is told of all the potential complications and alternatives to that procedure. It is then the patient's responsibility to ask any questions she may harbor and then, based on all this information, consent to or refuse the procedure. This book is like an informed consent for menopause. You will be presented with a great deal of information, yet the final decision on action is yours.

SECTION 1
LAYING THE
FOUNDATION

ℬ

THE HEALING TRIAD

"I'm falling apart, and I don't know how to put all the pieces back together."

Shelly was nearly at the end of her rope and sliding fast. She was an anxious woman in her late forties who was looking for answers and wanting them quickly.

"My biggest two problems are that I have no energy and absolutely no sex drive," Shelly told me. "Even when I do feel good, I would rather knit than make love. My husband likes sweaters, but not that much! This menopause stuff makes puberty look like a walk in the park!"

I was relieved that Shelly still had her sense of humor. She was going to need it! For Shelly to resolve her issues, she needed to approach her situation from three separate, yet related, directions. She had to look at her problems not as isolated afflictions but as interrelated experiences. This was her chance to explore solutions involving her mind, body, and spirit. Focusing solely on her physical symptoms and not addressing causes would doom her to failure.

As it turned out, Shelly was fatigued from her hypertension medication. She also suffered from painful intercourse, which led to her libido problems. Furthermore, during her initial exam, she revealed that an uncle had sexually abused her when she was eleven, and she had never been able to tell any family members about her trauma. She was a deeply religious woman but didn't see any connection between her current physical problems and her spiritual life.

The solutions to Shelly's problems were multiple. They involved not only changing her blood pressure medication and giving her estrogen to increase vaginal lubrication, but also extensive counseling from her pastor, who was a certified counselor. With the medical changes she felt physically great, but it was the spiritual and emotional work that helped her feel whole.

To become healed (whole), Shelly had to balance her body with her mind (beliefs, thoughts, and emotions) and her spirit (her relationship with God). To ignore any component of this healing triad would rob Shelly of true wellness.

Shelly's healing path began with an understanding that she was not defined by her maladies. She was a child of God, intrinsically healthy, who was temporarily out of balance.

Health for Shelly, and for each of us, is not just the absence of disease. It is much more than that. The word *health* originally meant "to make whole," and this embodies an accurate and biblical description of the term. A healthy person is one who strives for a balance among all the components of wellness.

Many in the healing professions focus exclusively on the health of the physical body. This is incomplete because it ignores the powerful influence of thoughts, emotions, and feelings on our health. We are, in many ways, what we think. This dualism of mind and body is more congruent with a true concept of healing and wholeness. However, limiting thinking to only these two parameters is still imperfect.

> A healthy body is a guest chamber for the soul, a sick body is a prison.
>
> —Francis Bacon

You may be in excellent physical health and mentally acute, yet you may still be in sorrowful pain. It is an elusive discomfort burrowed deep in your heart. It is a pain that arises from your innermost being, your soul. Indeed, you are struggling with the third component of wellness, that of the spirit. Being physically fit and mentally sharp is not enough. Only by filling your spiritual void can a balance be achieved. To fully realize your health potential, you must seek and feed this universal spiritual hunger. The Bible feeds this hunger with its guidance, wisdom, and practical advice.

There is an intimate connection among these three entities (mind, body, and spirit) that links their purpose. It is like a mobile hanging over a baby's crib. If you pull on one part of the mobile, all of the other parts move in response. So it is with your health. A change in your physical body will impact how you feel emotionally. It is hard to achieve balance and contentment in your physical and emotional health if your spiritual life is not vigorous.

COMFORT

There will come a time in your race through midlife that you experience pain and frustration. We all do; it is inevitable. During the dark times, you may ask yourself, *How can I best go on? What now? Why me?* The answers lie in your preparation. What is the foundation that supports you in hard times? What carries you those last few miles when you want so desperately to quit? Better yet, what is it that gives you the ability, confidence, and wisdom to confront the challenges of midlife and menopause? You prepare with applied knowledge, life experience, and faith.

You can run the race of life knowing that it will be fraught with ruts and roadblocks; however, you can be secure in knowing that you are not running alone. This is where physiology and medicines fall short. Pills and creams make lousy comforters. If you focus only on the mind and the body, you will miss the reassurance of the spirit. There is comfort, knowledge, and strength in the Word of God. Nowhere is this contentment better illustrated than in the twenty-third Psalm. . . . *even in menopause.* (The parentheses are my attempt to show lighthearted relevance.)

The Twenty-Third Psalm (Even in Menopause)

The Lord is my shepherd; I have all that I need. (I'm fat, fatigued, and fifty!)
He lets me rest in green meadows; (Even with hot flashes)
He leads me beside peaceful streams. (In the middle of night sweats)
He renews my strength. (When fatigue takes over)
He guides me along right paths, bringing honor to his name. (Showing me options)
Even when I walk through the darkest valley, I will not be afraid, for you are close beside me. (Depression cannot rule me.)
Your rod and your staff protect and comfort me. (Herbs and vitamins too)
You prepare a feast for me in the presence of my enemies. You honor me by anointing my head with oil. (Flaxseed, chamomile)
My cup overflows with blessings. (At least I am here to experience menopause—the other option is not so great.)
Surely your goodness and unfailing love will pursue me all the days of my life, and I will live in the house of the Lord forever. (Wrinkles and all)

MENOPAUSE EXPLOSION

The shelves at the local bookstore are bursting with how-to and how-not-to books on menopause. Menopause has come out of the closet! Celebrities are embracing their age (those who don't thrive on plastic surgery) and endorsing everything from bioidentical hormones to incontinence medicines. Just a few years back it was impossible to find any books solely devoted to menopause. Just asking the clerk or librarian brought smirks or hushed murmurs. "We don't have much on *that* subject, dear." It was as if you had to wear a giant scarlet *M* on your dress to signify you were a wayward menopausal woman seeking information and restitution. Gail Sheehy writes in her 1992 bestseller, *The Silent Passage*, "In trying to learn or talk about menopause, I found myself up against a powerful and mysterious taboo. My friends were adrift in the same fog of inexcusable ignorance. We couldn't help each other because none of us knew enough."[1] I think Ms. Sheehy would agree that "you've come a long way, baby" since then.

Now women march in the street "taking back" their menopause. (I never knew anyone took it away!) They proudly proclaim the sisterhood of aging as a dominant social force as the menopausal demographic explodes. It is important not to fall prey to the "spiritual feminism" that pervades some of this movement. The pendulum of awareness has swung so far that several women have commented that they feel guilty for not having menopausal problems! They are reflecting the wealth of negativism infecting the common perception of menopause. This is a monumental problem, as the dominant attitude in Western culture is both overtly and covertly one of menopause as a disease. The medical and pharmaceutical professions are largely guilty of perpetuating this myth. Traditional medical training still holds fast to the idea that menopause is an estrogen-deficiency disease. This is antiquated and hopefully will be expelled from our collective consciousness in the near future.

> As of this book's printing, Amazon.com lists well over 21,000 books with menopause in the title!

When menopause is discussed in the media, it is often presented in a less than attractive manner. It is much more sensational and newsworthy to talk about hardships, cancer-causing medicines, bad times, and evil hot-flash demons than it is to talk of joy, celebrations, and solutions. The tone of this discourse is similar to the way your sister-in-law may discuss her nightmarish labor. Inevitably the discussion is energized by the details of a seventy-two-hour descent into hell orchestrated by a nine-pound alien! This is not to belittle those who truly had difficult labors, but the stories tend to become embellished over time. You hear these stories because they are more interesting and dramatic. Few new moms droll on about their incredibly easy and quick delivery—it's just not as fascinating. With time you begin to unconsciously view labor as a terrific ordeal because you have been continually bombarded with tales of terror. Repetitive conditioning has also relegated menopause to the horror story hall of fame.

You don't hear the great success stories, and there are many. You don't hear about the huge number of women who have few complaints and breeze through the transition. Only 15 percent of women in menopause have severe symptoms.[2] But you only read and hear the tragedies and tribulations of those who struggle with menopausal madness. So as time passes and God grants you a midlife, all of these images come racing back. If the war stories are from an influential woman in your life (like the aunt who left you millions in her will), the negative impact can be immense. It is a good thing for women to feel open and free to discuss their menopausal experience, but be wary of the doomsayers.

RESOURCES

Books abound on the subject. The Internet, that hotbed of accurate and timely knowledge on the level of the *Enquirer*, has thousands of sites focusing exclusively on menopause and menopausal issues. The information superhighway is a good thing, but just as you wouldn't stop along the regular highway and pick up a dead skunk, be cautious not to pick up every bit of information you find on the Internet. Table 1 lists some great Internet sites that provide useful and valid information. View all resources with a critical eye. Even if it appears to be educational only, consider the source. Is there an agenda? Is there some hidden purpose in what you see and hear? Are they trying to sell you something?

TABLE 1: INTERNET SITES

www.guidetohormonehealth.com . . .	Your obvious first stop!
www.fatproofyourfamily.com . . .	My first book, a shameless promotion
www.menopause.org . . .	Web site of North American Menopause Society, a great starting place
www.herbs.org . . .	Excellent information and current research on herbal medicines
www.healthywomen.org . . .	Good starting point for general health issues for women
www.nof.org . . .	Home of the National Osteoporosis Foundation
www.menopause-online.com . . .	A balanced view of both traditional and nontraditional approaches

www.power-surge.com . . .	Power Surge newsletter, excellent site, lots of well-presented practical information
www.acog.org . . .	American College of Obstetricians and Gynecologists
www.webmd.com . . .	Good clearinghouse of non-biased information
www.healthy.net . . .	Good mix of traditional and nontraditional information on a variety of subjects

THE SELLING OF MENOPAUSE

Menopause has become the latest darling of Madison Avenue. It has not only come out of the closet, but it has leaped into the bank vault. Why? Because there is a great deal of money to be made! With the aging of the baby boomers, more women are entering menopause than at any other time in history. Women over sixty-five will soon be one of the fastest-growing segments of the population. This is a huge market, as many drug company executives are discovering. In 1997 it was estimated that 83 million Americans spent over 27 billion dollars on alternative health care.[3] Much of this cash flowed toward the purchase of herbs and vitamins, which are an important component of alternative approaches to menopause.

Google *menopause* and you get over 13 million listings!

The pharmaceutical industry in this country alone is a multibillion-dollar industry. Many companies that have a long history of developing only prescription medicines have now launched entire divisions devoted to over-the-counter drugs. They have targeted menopause because of the huge demographics, less regulation, lower liability, and fear of prescription hormones. Direct-to-consumer advertising has cluttered most media outlets praising the latest breakthroughs in "natural" menopause management. Various pharmaceutical giants promote "menopause relief formulas" and "female remedies."

The upside to this increased attention to herbal medicines is that it may spawn additional efficacy and safety research in the United States. My realistic, cynical self believes, however, that minimal work will be done with these substances since no one company has a monopoly on their production.

Simply follow the money! A warranted fear is that the poor quality and unpredictable reliability of products from unregulated manufacturers will throw a veil of impropriety over the entire industry. Thus natural medicine manufacturers must police their own to guarantee quality and consistency in their products, or educated consumers will shun their goods.

Menopause has become a major money-generating industry. One of the most prescribed drugs of all time is Premarin, an estrogen replacement tablet. In 2001, this drug generated around two billion dollars in sales for its manufacturer, Wyeth-Ayerst.[4] Menopause is a multifaceted economic diamond ready to be mined. The expansive market base that is largely untapped (remember only 17 percent of eligible women take hormone replacement therapy) is being courted.

A study by researchers at the Stanford Center for Research in Disease Prevention estimated that "the U.S. pharmaceutical industry spent $12.7 billion promoting its products in 1998." Premarin was one of the top 5 drugs studied.[5]

Pick up any magazine targeting women and you will be accosted with ads for hormone replacement therapy. If the publication's demographics are specifically targeted to the over-thirty-five woman, there will likely be at least one ad spewing the estrogen necessity fallacy. Notice the subtle nature of the ads. Almost all appeal to vanity. They scream, "Look good, feel good, and stay sexy!" Ads may not state it overtly, but if you dissect the intent and presentation, they inevitably make direct or indirect reference to physical appearance, mental functioning, or sexuality. This is not by accident; it is by design.

Hormone replacement was originally promoted years ago as a cosmetic-like substance. It was a way to keep you "feminine forever." That attitude has persisted in marketing departments throughout the drug and supplement industries. They understand that your desire to stay young and thwart aging is what will sell their products. Granted, they also emphasize the long-term benefits such as osteoporosis prevention, yet the subliminal message is "use hormones and stay beautiful." I find it ironic that Hollywood, so long a bastion of "young at all costs," now embraces this market with celebrities touting the benefits of hormones. Again, follow the money.

With the explosion of popular interest in menopause, the drug companies have shifted their advertising strategy to focus on the consumer.

They realize that their customer is no longer the physician who prescribes their drug but the consumer who goes to the doctor demanding the new pill she saw advertised on TV. The companies understand the relative laziness of the consumer; therefore, they aggressively define both the problem and the solution. Needless to say, they provide a solution that promotes their products. What the drug companies have effectively done is defined menopause as a disease that needs to be treated. This attitude is wrong and must be reversed.

To be a wise consumer, you must be critical of the information you receive. Evaluate the source. This is not to suggest that all information disseminated by drug manufacturers is suspect. Some generic facts and figures are helpful. However, companies are in the business of selling, and most information they distribute will be designed to sell their products.

The marketing of menopause also reflects the differences in how a doctor and patient may view this transition. You are most likely to view menopause as a time of symptoms and changes that need attention, and your interest and actions are more reactive to symptoms. Many physicians, on the other hand, continue to approach menopause as an estrogen-deficiency disease and prescribe hormones primarily for potential health benefits. For them, symptomatic treatment is a secondary gain. Unfortunate to this line of thought are the numerous recent studies that suggest long-term hormone use has minimal preventive indications. (I will expand on the pros and cons in a following chapter.)

Menopause is no more an estrogen-deficiency disease than a headache is a Tylenol-deficiency disease! There are those in the medical community who believe strongly that every woman, with few exceptions, should be prescribed hormones! That is a dangerous philosophy. God didn't create you with a built-in obsolescence. You were not designed to automatically "fall apart" at age fifty-one, as some would have you think. This biomedical view of menopause as a disease has galvanized the marketing of menopause. If the public recognizes this transition as a medical affliction, then it only makes sense that it must be treated. And how do we do that in this country? Drugs!

As more and more women are clamoring for other approaches, the slick marketers are saying, "Sure, we have herbs and vitamins. Take those [made by us] if you don't like our estrogen products." In fact, many large pharmaceutical companies that manufacture hormones have bought smaller companies that make and distribute natural remedies for menopause to tap in to this growing market.

Many of the advertisements for estrogen, and much of the lay literature, subliminally project the concept that if you don't use estrogen you will inevitably end up as a wrinkled, sexless, old, dried-up woman. This is not only untrue, but it is also an insult to women. You can live a vibrant, healthy, long life using a variety of techniques, foods, activities, and medicines if you so choose. The use of hormones is not the criteria for health, longevity, or physical beauty.

Many physicians and health-care personnel are becoming more supportive of the concept of a transitional approach to menopause, an approach that is cognizant of the normalcy of the change and recognizes the importance of choice and responsibility. This is the approach this book will embrace.

THE FOUR A'S

Many of the lifestyle choices you make, such as diet and exercise, can dramatically affect your menopausal experience. Given average life expectancy, you may live a third of all your days in postmenopause. It is not a time to be complacent or anxious. It is a time, a season, to rejoice and celebrate what God has provided.

What is the prescription for midlife miracles? The four A's: attitude, aptitude, action, and apothecary.

Attitude

What we believe is our reality, what we *know* is our truth. In Paul's letter to the Romans, he tells us to become new people by changing our attitudes. Believe in the celebration of menopause. Be glad for midlife. It is the end of reproduction, but not of production. Every action begins with a thought, and you are the only one who controls your thoughts.

> The greatest discovery of my generation is that a human being can alter his life by altering his attitudes of mind.
>
> —William James

Aptitude

Educate yourself; learn your options. Ask questions, talk to others, and take responsibility. "Fear of the Lord is the beginning of knowledge, but fools despise wisdom and discipline" (Proverbs 1:7 NIV).

Action

There are two levels of action. First, act on what you know. The key to any person's success, whether in business or in the home, is taking action. A great idea is only great if acted upon. There is nothing sadder than a good idea that dies from loneliness or lack of attention. You can design a game plan, but if you don't execute it, failure is inevitable.

Second, get off your behind and get moving! Exercise is the fountain of youth and a cleansing activity for mind, body, and spirit. There is commotion where there is no motion! Exercise is not an option but a requirement if you are to aspire to good health in menopause and beyond.

Apothecary

Apothecary is a historical name for someone who prepares and dispenses medicines to doctors and patients — a role now served by a pharmacist. Because apothecaries worked closely with herbal and chemical ingredients, it is noted that they may be regarded as a precursor of the modern sciences of chemistry and pharmacology.

Some of you may remember the old-time drugstores known as apothecaries. Not only did they sell prescription medicines, but they had a lunch counter, a place where you could get the best salves and balms, and often a pharmacist who would jump at the chance to give you an opinion . . . about anything! The idea of foods and herbs as medicines will be explored (as will the other A's) in the following chapters.

DEFINITIONS

Before we go further, let's define some important terms so we are all thinking alike. (That's a scary thought, all of us thinking alike!)

Menopause is simply a cessation of periods. That's it. And this can only be identified in retrospect. In other words, you don't know it was your last period until six months have gone by and you have had no others. Technically, you have to be without a period for a year to qualify as menopausal; however, chances are good you're menopausal if you go without one for six months or more. The average age for natural menopause is fifty-one.

Surgical menopause is when your ovaries are removed prior to the time they would normally cease functioning. This is most commonly done at the time of a hysterectomy; however, the ovaries are not removed automatically at every hysterectomy. A hysterectomy removes only the uterus and cervix. The uterus doesn't have a hormonal production role as do the ovaries, so simply removing the uterus does not cause surgical menopause even though the periods cease. If you have a hysterectomy *and* removal of your ovaries at thirty-four, for example, then you are surgically menopausal at that point.

Don't be confused by the often-used terminology *total hysterectomy* or *partial hysterectomy*. When people use these terms, they are labeling a total hysterectomy as one in which the ovaries are removed, and a partial hysterectomy as one in which the ovaries remain. This is an important distinction. It is the removal of the ovaries that creates surgical menopause. Simply removing the uterus (the partial hysterectomy, in slang terms) will not make you surgically menopausal since your ovaries are intact and still going full blast. I would encourage you to drop the *total* versus *partial* terminology and actually describe what is removed.

Perimenopause is a more useful term in assessing symptoms. This is the time frame around menopause. It can vary in its length and onset and is actually defined by the presence of symptoms. There is no set age or time that marks perimenopause. It is as individual as your own experience. In other words, if you are forty-two and having severe hormonal hot flashes, you may be in perimenopause. On the other hand, you may not have any symptoms or warnings before your periods cease. My mother is such a soul. To this day she can't understand what the uproar over menopause is all about. She had (and still has) absolutely no symptoms! Nothing. *Nada.* She would rather I devote myself to real problems like remembering her birthday and calling on Sundays!

It is useful to use the term *postmenopausal* to describe the time after the periods cease. Many will continue to use *perimenopausal* to refer to this time, but this confuses people. Simply stated, perimenopause is the time leading up to menopause, and postmenopause is the time after the cessation of menses. This book treats perimenopause and premenopause interchangeably.

Premenstrual syndrome (PMS) is a clinically identifiable syndrome with a physiological basis. PMS symptoms may appear for the first time in midlife, and often PMS and perimenopausal symptoms are confused. Telling a woman in the throes of PMS that she is just experiencing a few hormonal fluctuations is like calling a hurricane a breath of fresh air. I take it seriously, and so should you. More on this later.

Estrogen is the predominant female hormone. It can take several different chemical forms. It is the most abundant hormone of the triad that affects women and their cycles. The other two major hormones are *progesterone* and *testosterone*. Progesterone is the hormone that is predominantly secreted either after ovulation or in the first part of pregnancy. It is an important component of hormone replacement treatment when a woman has *not* had a hysterectomy. Testosterone is commonly referred to as the "male hormone" largely because it is the hormone that predominates in the male system. It is produced by women in lower concentrations and plays an important role in sexuality and well-being.

Another term you may hear is *climacteric*. This refers to the time around menopause, and many equate this term with perimenopause. Often it is used to include both pre- and postmenopausal scenarios. It actually is used very little today, yet you may come across it in older literature.

Hormone replacement therapy (HRT) is the use of prescription medicines, both synthetic and bioidentical, to treat menopausal symptoms. They commonly include various mixtures of estrogen, progesterone, and testosterone (much more on this later).

Bioidentical or "natural" hormones are prescription medicines that mimic what your body naturally produces. They are usually plant derived but are still manufactured in the lab. They are natural in the sense that they are identical in chemical composition to the hormones produced in the ovaries. There is an ongoing debate in the health world as to their advantages and disadvantages as compared to synthetic hormones. Don't confuse these prescription medicines with herbs or other nutraceuticals.

ACTION CHALLENGE

Starting today, shift your focus from one of worry and lack to one of praise and abundance. God has a plan and, no matter how old, how sick, how crabby, or how stubborn you are, that plan can be realized. The fulfillment of that plan depends solely on two forces: you and God. My money says God will do his part; your challenge is to do yours. Start today by making the decision to think differently.

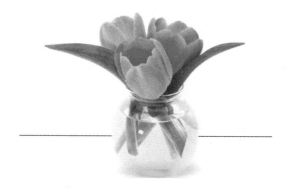

COMPLEMENTARY MEDICINE AND THE BIBLE

Sue Ellen was confused mentally and spiritually. She was a bright, articulate mother of two who was struggling with her emotions and her body. She came to my office on a Friday afternoon, complaining mainly of fatigue. "I'm always so tired, and I mean all the time! I sleep well at night, but by midday I am just dragging. Dr. Eaker, I'm too young to be this old!"

We talked about her physical symptoms, and then I did a thorough physical exam. As we talked it became apparent that she had read some books on herbs and fatigue—she was a take-charge person—but was bothered by the New Age philosophy that seemed to pervade what she read. She didn't want to take drugs to improve her energy level, so she sought more natural approaches. She was a devout Christian and said, "I have to wade through a lot of weird-sounding mumbo jumbo to get to the information on alternative approaches that I want. Is this okay, or should I avoid this kind of stuff altogether?"

Sue Ellen is not alone in her confusion. Is alternative medicine unchristian? Can a woman use herbs and vitamins and not compromise her religious beliefs? The answer to these and other questions depends on an accurate understanding of the terms. Along with a meteoric rise in interest in menopause has come a resurgence in "natural" and "alternative" approaches to midlife and its changes. It is important to define these terms to avoid misunderstandings.

It is easy to "mis-hear" when ambiguous and unclear terms are used. Medicine is buried in jargon, and one of the biggest complaints you may have with your doctor is that he talks in medical speak.

Let me attempt to translate the medical speak into normal speak. A natural substance is anything that occurs *by design* in nature or in your body. Therefore, it does not include synthetic chemicals or man-altered medications. An equivalent term is *bioidentical*. You will encounter this term often today as it has been popularized by the press and celebrity endorsers. For purposes of this discussion, I will use the terms *natural hormones* and *bioidentical hormones* synonymously.

For example, progesterone cream contains the exact chemical substance that is in your body. This is a natural, or bioidentical, substance. Even though the actual product is made in a laboratory through a process of chemical reactions, the final substance is one that is naturally occurring in the healthy human. Conversely, Provera, or medroxyprogesterone acetate, is a progesterone-like substance created in the lab to facilitate its oral use. This is not a natural substance. Nowhere in your system will you find a naturally occurring molecule of medroxyprogesterone acetate.

NATURAL ISN'T ALWAYS SAFER

This definition of *natural* is extremely inclusive. This implies nothing about effectiveness, safety, side effects, or cost. It also does not imply who can or who cannot utilize or recommend such substances. We serve a God of abundance, but to discover that abundance we have to do our homework. There is an innate obligation and responsibility to understand and explore what God has provided. God knows our needs and provides for them through a variety of channels.

Common definitions of "natural"

- ๛ Existing in or produced by nature; not artificial or imitation
- ๛ Existing in or in conformity with nature or the observable world; neither supernatural nor magical
- ๛ Functioning or occurring in a normal way; lacking abnormalities or deficiencies
- ๛ Unthinking
- ๛ Prompted by (or as if by) instinct
- ๛ Being unprocessed or manufactured using only simple or minimal processes (used especially of commodities)
- ๛ Someone regarded as certain to succeed
- ๛ Related by blood, not adopted
- ๛ Being talented through inherited qualities
- ๛ Lifelike, free from artificiality

Substances should not be universally acknowledged as healthy by virtue of their "natural" label. Our family was at the beach several summers ago, and my wife asked me to take a picture of our two little girls (then five and three) for a Christmas card. We wandered through the sand dunes until we found a beautiful display of flowers, sand, and surf that would appropriately highlight my little angels. They picked a couple of the pretty flowers (at my request) to hold to attempt to emulate the pictures I had seen from much more qualified photographers.

After I had taken what I was sure was a Pulitzer Prize photo, an older couple watching us nearby casually commented that the pretty flowers our girls were holding were an extremely poisonous variety that would be very harmful if gnawed on by our young models! Needless to say, I quickly snatched the flowers from their hands and, as they burst into tears, I tried to explain to them why the pretty flowers were not good to play with. To this day my daughter delights in telling everyone about the time Daddy tried to poison her! My point is that just because something is labeled as "natural" doesn't mean it is necessarily healthy or useful. Not all of God's creation was meant to be appreciated in the same way!

A common misperception about natural products is that they have few side effects and they are safer than prescription medicines. But many herbal preparations, when ingested in improper amounts, may produce marked complications. An example is the herb Ma Huang, which is in a number of the natural weight loss products. This herb has been associated with heart arrhythmias (irregular heartbeats) and hypertension. Another example involves the fat-soluble vitamins A, D, E, and K, which can build up to toxic levels if taken in high enough doses over an extended time. You can get too much of a good thing. Combining some "natural" substances can also be harmful. Their side effects can be synergistic and counterproductive.

An issue rapidly coming to the forefront is the combination of prescription medicines and herbal treatments. One survey stated that over 15 million people combined one or more medications with one or more herbal products. This same survey asserted that about 60 percent of people using herbal products don't discuss them with their doctors.[1] How many times have you gone to the doctor and been asked to fill out forms listing your medications? Inevitably you leave off your Saint-John's-wort or your black cohosh, simply because you don't consider these medications.

Potential interactions with common herbal medicines

- ∞ Echinacea may cause inflammation of the liver if used with certain other medications, such as anabolic steroids, methotrexate, or others.

- ∞ Ephedra may interact with certain antidepressant medications or certain high blood pressure medications to cause dangerous elevation in blood pressure or heart rate. It could cause death in certain individuals.

- ∞ Garlic, ginger, and Ginkgo may increase bleeding, especially in patients already taking certain anti-clotting medications.

- ∞ Kava may increase the effects of certain anti-seizure medications and/or prolong the effects of certain anesthetics. It can enhance the effects of alcohol. It may increase the risk of suicide for people with certain types of depression.

- ∞ Saint-John's-wort may prolong the effect of certain anesthetic agents.

- ∞ Valerian may increase the effects of certain anti-seizure medications or prolong the effects of certain anesthetic agents.

This is of great concern because there are some combinations that can be dangerous, especially before surgery.

As you explore your options, share your discoveries with your doctor or pharmacist. Keep an accurate and current list of all prescription medications, and don't be hesitant to discuss your use of alternative therapies with your doctor. It is information that they need to know.

A healthy balance requires initiating a dialogue with your doctor about any possible drug interactions. Thankfully, there is a great margin of safety with most natural products, but be smart. Using natural substances is not an excuse to put your brain on a shelf.

Many of us know that using herbs and vitamins can be quite challenging. Sorting through the hundreds of brands and dosages and staying on a consistent regimen takes effort. If you are looking for a quick, easy fix to your symptoms with herbs, you will be disappointed, because a long-term successful regimen, whether hormone replacement therapy or naturals, involves commitment and persistence. Clearly, there is no one option that works for everyone.

What does alternative medicine mean to you? Many women have a preconceived idea of that term's definition. In other words, they know what it means cognitively, but there is inevitably an emotional rider to this understanding. Don't let prior beliefs be impediments to understanding legitimate choices and options. Expand your point of reference.

Most people view alternative approaches as any therapy outside the mainstream of current medically accepted treatment and diagnostic modalities. During a discussion with a refined older lady about alternative methods of dealing with menopausal complaints, I noticed a look of apprehension on her face. When I commented on this, she blurted out, "You're not going to get naked and burn incense are you?" Images of crystals and Eastern mystics clouded her perception of what alternative medicine means.

ALTERNATIVE APPROACHES

The definition of *alternative* is totally dependent on the era and culture in which it is used. Currently, acceptable medical treatment is defined by both the governing bodies of national associations and by the local laws and customs where it is practiced. Traditional and nontraditional medical practices are culturally dependent. They can and do change with time. Many thought Edward Jenner was insane when he proposed preventing smallpox by injecting a similar virus from cows into humans. There were cartoons that depicted people receiving the smallpox vaccine and watching in horror as a cow head or udder sprouted from their necks; however, Jenner's proposal set the stage for modern immunizations!

What is now thought of as state-of-the-art may at a later date be viewed as archaic, and the reverse is true. However, there are some universal and constant truths. What the Bible says about health and long life is still applicable today! It is as valid now as it was two millennia ago. This testifies to the eternal truths the Bible teaches. Because God is living, transcendent, and unchanging, you can trust him to help you now, just as he helped in past generations.

COMPLEMENTARY MEDICINE

A more inclusive and accurate term for understanding legitimate alternative treatment is *complementary medicine*. The connotation is that this is a different approach than the traditional; however, the two can be simultaneously employed. *Alternative* implies exclusivity whereas *complementary* implies inclusiveness, and that is more consistent with the belief system we are working with. The term *alternative medicine* is unfortunately fused to a particular philosophical and pseudo-spiritual movement. The New Age movement has been identified with some alternative medical practices because of a few shared terms and techniques. In reality these associations are in-

Traditional Chinese medicine, often the darling of alternative practitioners, lauds acupuncture as one of its most successful remedies for numerous ailments. "The general theory of acupuncture is based on the premise that there are patterns of energy flow (Qi) through the body that are essential for health. Disruptions of this flow are believed to be responsible for disease. The acupuncturist [claims to correct] imbalances of flow at identifiable points close to the skin." However, The National Council Against Health Fraud has concluded that acupuncture is an unproven modality of treatment, and research during the past 20 years has not demonstrated that acupuncture is effective against any disease.[2]

valid, although it is incumbent on the individual to separate the spiritual foundation from the scientific validity. Be careful not to issue a blanket condemnation of alternative therapies based on incorrect associations.

The term *New Age* is fraught with emotional baggage, and it is usually misunderstood. It brings about a negative guttural response in Christian circles based on its heretical overtones. To many Christians, New Age spirituality is a major affront to their beliefs, and I agree with their apprehension, based on my own interpretation of what New Age means. I believe the vast majority of practices labeled "New Age" are deceptive, ineffective, and dangerous. However, there is little new in the New Age, and I don't see this as a major problem in the areas we will be discussing. A good rule of thumb is to avoid anything labeled "New Age" as it is often pseudo-spiritual propaganda. It is possible that you may miss some information, but usually the good stuff is found in other resources. Therefore, in this book, less traditional approaches will be labeled as "complementary" treatments. Remember to separate the science and the philosophy when appropriate.

THE BIBLE AS A USER'S MANUAL

What does the Bible say about designs for living, and how does this apply to midlife and menopause? Both the Old and New Testaments contain specific and practical guidance on foods, moods, exercise, prayer, stress, anxiety, herbs, attitude, and healing. The Bible not only gives guidelines to emulate, it also presents specific examples and role models.

The women of the Bible serve as role models for today's woman. Virginia Owens, in her book *Daughters of Eve*, asks,

> How much has life really changed for women? Are there, in fact, gendered propensities that persist over time, threads that run through time and across cultures revealing essential patterns? Are we, even after centuries of change, still "sisters under the skin" with the Middle Eastern, North African, and Mediterranean women who span the biblical pages? Do their fears and sorrows, hopes and joys connect with ours? If we paid attention to them, would they have anything significant to say to us?[3]

She then proceeds to answer those penetrating and relevant questions with a resounding "yes" by showing in excellent detail how women in the Bible speak clearly and loudly to the women of today. Such unforgettable personalities as Ruth, Naomi, Mary, Martha, and Hannah provide excellent examples of God's guidance for living and believing.

It flows logically that the greatest how-to book ever written provides a plethora of practical mentors, and you will see how some of these women's stories illustrate God's plan for a successful journey through menopause.

MENOPAUSE AND OLD AGE

As we have said, menopause is the end of reproduction but not the end of production. Many of the negative feelings in the Western world toward menopause arise from its close association with aging. At seminars around the country I always ask the audience to play the "free association" game. When I say the word *menopause*, inevitably someone will yell out "old" or "aging," and it usually gets worse from there.

Whether we like it or not, we still live in a youth-oriented society. Mirroring modern culture, the advertising industry reflects the desirability of youth. Conversely, aging is portrayed as a horrid condition to be avoided at all cost. You may think this is an exaggeration, yet look closely at magazine ads or TV commercials. The obsession with being or looking young is evident.

Some will resort to ridiculous gyrations to retain at least the physical appearance of youth. One gross misperception is that a physical change will be translated into an emotional rebirth: If we look young, we will feel young. Those who have attempted to keep pace with a granddaughter on a mall outing realize that looking young and feeling young are not always compatible. No matter how young we think we are, physical laws dictate that there comes a time when our knees buckle but our belts won't. Some say you have reached that mature age when your back goes out more than you do. For those who are feeling a bit dismayed at this reality, remember the words as written in Isaiah: "I will be your God throughout your lifetime—until your hair is white with age. I made you, and I will care for you. I will carry you along and save you" (Isaiah 46:4).

Samuel Johnson wrote, "He that would pass the latter part of his life with honor and decency, must, when he is young, consider that he shall one day be old; and remember, when he is old, that he has once been young."[4] The problem in midlife and menopause is that the invoices from the purchases of our youth come due at this time.

DON'T BE A VICTIM

"Today's older Americans are very different from their predecessors, living longer, having lower rates of disability, achieving higher levels of education and less often living in poverty. In fact, recent demographic estimates indicate that seniors comprise 47% of the leisure travel market or 144 million room nights per year. Today's seniors are relatively active, healthy, and young at heart. They control half of the nation's discretionary income and are America's fastest-growing age group. The U.S. Federal Reserve Board reports that the over-50 age group now controls 77% of the nation's financial holdings worth about $800 billion; represents about 35% of the total U.S. population; and accounts for 42% of after-tax income."[5]

One area where complementary approaches and biblical teachings coincide is in assessing the impact of our thoughts on our physical well-being. Proverbs 14:30 says, "A peaceful heart leads to a healthy body; jealousy is like cancer in the bones." What we believe often becomes our reality, so it is understandable that menopause has developed a negative aura in Western society. It is not that way in other cultures. Social anthropologists find that negative symptoms of menopause are almost nonexistent in cultures where aging is revered and respected! The word for "hot flash" doesn't even exist in Japan. A study done a few years ago compared the symptoms of menopause cross-culturally and found that the single greatest factor that influenced the intensity and variety of symptoms of menopause was the individual's perception of aging![6] This is exciting information in that it shifts responsibility from the external to the internal. In other words, menopause doesn't have to be something that happens to you; it is something you can influence. You don't change the basic physiology, but you train your body to respond to changes differently. Instead of simply reacting to symptoms, you can train your mind and body to minimize the occurrence of symptoms!

You can have a marked impact on your menopausal experience by changing your thoughts. You can go from a victim mentality to a belief system that promotes control over your physical and emotional destiny. This is a revelation to those who have been inundated with messages that this thing called menopause is inevitably bad—and worse, that you are powerless to do anything about it. There is control; there are choices. This time in your life is a joyous one and can be celebrated.

INTEGRATION

If there is something unhealthy or troublesome in your thoughts, it will, in some way, impact your physical body. Many have experienced situations where our thoughts and emotions were the direct precursors to physical symptoms. There is a fascinating branch of science called psychoneuro-immunology that studies the effects of thoughts, feelings, and emotions on the immune system. In this age of AIDS awareness, much is known about the importance of a properly functioning immune system. This area of study has shown conclusively that strong emotional states can have a profound influence on how, for example, white blood cells produce antibodies that fight disease. Being anxious or upset can lead to physical illness! Anger has been shown to impede the white blood cells' ability to ward off invading viruses. This may explain why colds and runny noses proliferate during times of high stress. In his book *Health and Medicine in the Methodist Tradition*, E. Brooks Holifield writes, "A diseased brain could produce delirium of spirit, disordered nerves could engender distempered thoughts, and obstructed circulation could create spiritual temptations."[7]

In 1975 Robert Ader and Nicholas Cohen at the University of Rochester coined the term psychoneuroimmunology while working with rats and their immune system. They used sugar water and a powerful nausea-initiating drug to study the rats' immune system response to stress.

This miraculous interdependence serves as a natural guardian of health. Conversely, it can also serve as a source of multiple stresses and imbalances. All menopausal experiences have an impact on not only your physical body but also your emotions, thoughts, and feelings, as well as your walk with God.

GOD'S PLAN

God wants you to be healthy. He cares for your natural body, which he created, as he does the spirit. God wants you to use common sense *and* medical science to achieve a balance in mind, soul, and body. But just as menopause is a unique experience for each one of you, so the way God guides you toward health may be different. God may lead you to certain foods or exercises that are tremendously effective for treating a specific problem, yet those same choices may be ineffective or even harmful for another person. The challenge is to take the knowledge available to you and prayerfully consider its application to your situation. God will not let you down. He designed us to be healthy, vibrant beings, and he provides us with the necessities to achieve this optimal balance of mind, body, and spirit. Patch Adams, a well-known physician and clown, says that health is a happy, vibrant life, doing the most with what you have, with delight.

Why is it important that you take care of your body and its needs? Should you assume that God will provide the needed healing for all of your ills or symptoms? Is it right to use medical science in helping with your maladies? Look at 1 Corinthians 6:19–20: "Don't you realize that your body is the temple of the Holy Spirit, who lives in you and was given to you by God? You do not belong to yourself, for God bought you with a high price. So you must honor God with your body." This does not simply say it would be nice to promote a healthy body; it is a command to honor God with your body. Paul is specifically referring to sexuality and morality in these verses, yet the applications are broader. The implied message is that to let your body fall into disrepair is to dishonor its Creator. You *must* honor God by how you take care of your body. It houses the sacred.

God always provides the mechanisms to fulfill his commands. This is consistent throughout the Bible. Your choice is whether to act on these instructions or to ignore them. It is never too late to make that choice. You may be wondering whether exercise and good nutrition can help you now if you have been neglectful in the past. You may feel a sense of hopelessness because of previous failures at living a healthy lifestyle. The endless diets, the unused gym memberships, and rampant obesity all contribute to this "What's the use?" mentality. These experiences definitely color your present behaviors, but God is an awesome God! With the proper motivation, action, education, and prayerful consideration of his desires for your health, you can overcome any obstacle.

ACHIEVING WHOLENESS

Remember, as followers of Jesus and believers of God's Word, we must tend to our bodies as well as our minds and spirits. We must honor God with our bodies, and we must use any means available to achieve health (wholeness). For you this may mean new and better dietary choices or starting an exercise program. This may mean using hormone replacement therapy or vitamins and dietary supplements. This may mean taking time to pray or to meditate to reduce stress.

The intentional will of God is that people remain healthy, *yet you must do your part*. It's up to you to make healthy lifestyle decisions. You cannot abdicate your responsibility. Being a Christian demands that you be accountable for your health practices. Being a Christian does not mean putting your brain or body on autopilot.

TAKING RESPONSIBILITY

There is a strong call for personal responsibility in making these choices. Much of the disease and poor health experienced today is generated from unhealthy lifestyle choices. If you analyze the leading causes of morbidity and mortality in the United States, you find that many lifestyle illnesses, such as obesity and heart disease, populate the leading indices.

You must take responsibility for using information, education, and action to facilitate your intrinsically healthy state. You cannot change the natural consequences of your actions. If you smoke, you dramatically increase your chances of lung cancer. God does not send lung cancer to you as punishment for smoking; it is the natural result of a conscious choice to abuse your body.

This concept of personal responsibility applies to menopausal changes. If you listen and obey God's words and take action to implement what you hear, you will find the fruits of your labors to be abundant.

Does this mean devout Christians don't become ill? Of course not. Anyone who uses that argument is missing the point. Simply being a Christian does not exclude you from the sickness and mishaps of a world bound by natural laws and consequences. Bad things happen to good people. However, you can control a major portion of your health by making wise choices.

You can also control your response to illness. In his book *Tuesdays with Morrie*, Mitch Albom writes about Morrie Shwartz, a favorite college mentor struck with Lou Gehrig's disease.

> What impressed me about Morrie was the honest acceptance of his illness and his exuberance to continue to live each day. He was reduced to total paralysis by this horrible disease yet his mind flourished and he cherished each day he was alive. Close to his death he said, "So many people walk around with a meaningless life. They seem half-asleep, even when they are busy doing things that seem important. This is because they are chasing the wrong things. The way you get meaning into your life is to devote yourself to loving others, devote yourself to the community around you, and devote yourself to creating something that gives you purpose and meaning."[8]

When Mitch asked him about his disease, Morrie replied, "It's only horrible if you see it that way. It's horrible to watch my body slowly wilt away to nothing. But it is also wonderful because of all the time I get to say good-bye. Not everyone is so lucky!"[9]

Health is a harmony of mind, body, and spirit. You can be ill physically yet still be whole in mind and spirit. When one part of the healing triad is broken, the others can provide support for a while.

RUNNING TO WIN

Menopause can be compared to a footrace. A marathon is a painful yet exhilarating experience. There is no escaping the fact that at some point in a 26.2-mile course you are going to feel pain. The question every marathon runner asks in every race is, "Do I have the will to go on?"

Some of us pose that question earlier in the race than others, but even world-class runners at some point say to themselves, "Is it worth it?" Your approach to menopause and the years beyond is much like a marathon. You spend the first fifty or so years of life preparing for the event. You learn, you train, you experience life. All this follows you to the race. No one arrives at the start line without the sum of their previous life experience with them. Just as in a race, much of how you "perform" during menopause is dependent on your preparation.

> About 450,000 Americans (40% female) ran marathons in 2002.

Most athletes will tell you that your training, education, and attitude going into the event are more important than the actual race. If you prepare properly, you have no fear. That is not to say that the race will not be challenging, but because of your preparation, the apprehension will evaporate and you will face the struggle with a sense of joy and confidence. At this point the race becomes a celebration. Similarly, if you prepare properly in mind, body, and spirit, menopause will be a celebration.

ACTION CHALLENGE

Take time to study Scripture, particularly as it applies to health and wellness. Use a concordance and look up verses that deal with health and sickness and see how these apply to your life.

SECTION 2

IS IT MENTAL PAUSE
OR MENOPAUSE?

❧

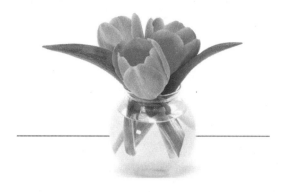

THE PERPLEXING PERIMENOPAUSE

A wise crone once said, "The only thing you can count on is that things will always change!" Change is one of the absolutes. Daily change gives life both its challenges and its flavor. The critical question we confront every day is, "How am I going to deal with both the little and the not-so-little changes?" President Jimmy Carter said, "What is life if not adjustment to different times, to our changing circumstances, and to each other?"[1]

Midlife and menopause are defined by change. In fact, when we capitalize the words *The Change*, most people immediately recognize the reference to menopause. Menopause is the "mother of all change."

To fully comprehend the nature of this transition, we must examine the time known as the perimenopause. It is the dress rehearsal for the big show. Some refer to this time as the climacteric, or premenopause. I prefer perimenopause because this is a more accurate characterization of the sequence of events. Besides, climacteric sounds funny, and everyone has trouble pronouncing it!

BIOLOGY 101

Most symptoms will begin, if at all, during this perimenopausal time. So the operative word here is *change*. Your body is changing, your emotions are changing, and your environment is changing. Let's begin learning how to take charge and make this change a celebration. The first step is understanding the physical changes that begin the process.

The female reproductive system is a miraculous creation. It is a complex, integrated, perfectly designed collection of organs, hormones, and tissues. There is no better example

> One human brain generates more electrical impulses in a single day than all of the world's telephones.

of how you are "fearfully and wonderfully made" (Psalm 139:14 NIV). The intricate interaction of all its parts overshadows any man-made creation and gives overwhelming evidence for intelligence and purpose in design.

The reproductive/endocrine system can be thought of as a three-story house. On the top floor sits the pituitary gland. This marble-sized structure at the base of the brain acts as the controller of the system. It sends out hormonal signals to the second story, the ovaries, and tells them to grow follicles that contain eggs. These developing follicles eventually respond to the pituitary's signals to stimulate ovulation. The ovaries, in addition to supporting and nourishing the developing eggs, secrete several hormones of their own, mainly estrogen, progesterone, and testosterone. The estrogen and progesterone act on the first story, the uterus, and lead to the buildup of the uterine lining and its eventual shedding, which is the monthly period. This cycle is repeated every twenty-eight to thirty-two days, unless one of the eggs meets up with a friendly sperm. If it is love at first sight, then the fertilized egg sets up a chain of events that leads to the uterine lining saying, "Hey, come on in and stay awhile—nine months to be exact."

As you age, the number of follicles in the ovary capable of developing into viable eggs decreases. At birth a woman has the greatest number of eggs she will ever possess. As the number of available eggs decreases, there is a concurrent decrease in active ovulations. These cycles are called anovulatory cycles, and they are significant because they can lead to missed or irregular periods.

A balance between estrogen and progesterone is required for the normal development and subsequent shedding of the uterine lining. Ovulation is the regulator of this balance. If ovulation stops, then the normal cycle is disrupted. This is basically what happens in perimenopause. The ovaries are ovulating less and less frequently, and this leads to a disruption of the normal cycles, and in turn to a change in the production of both estrogen and progesterone. As the estrogen levels decrease, there is minimal stimulation for the uterine lining to grow. So there comes a point where the periods cease. Presto, menopause!

These changes don't happen overnight. I'll never forget a scene from the '70s TV show *All in the Family*. Edith is going through "The Change," and Archie is becoming quite frustrated with her hot flashes and moodiness. At one point he grabs Edith and tosses her in a chair and says, "Okay, Edith, you have exactly three minutes to get over this menopause thing!"

It doesn't happen that way. These are slow processes that often occur over months or years. That is why perimenopause is such a nebulous term with no set guidelines for duration; each of you are different.

> Perimenopause is a process similar to puberty: It doesn't happen overnight. For many women, perimenopause can last anywhere from 5 to 15 years.

PMS OR PERIMENOPAUSE?

A major source of bewilderment during this time is distinguishing between PMS and perimenopause. The confusion often arises because the type and severity of symptoms can be similar in PMS and perimenopause, and they both occur commonly in a woman's early forties. PMS and perimenopause are rooted in hormonal changes, yet they are two separate entities, and therefore the treatments are very different. The causes of each are distinct, yet the end results (symptoms) can be almost identical.

PMS is real. It is not in your head. It does not stand for Punishing Men Slowly! For years women have been maligned, ridiculed, and told, "It's just that time of the month." What we (and by "we," I mean the predominantly male medical establishment) didn't understand was categorized as imaginary or unproven. Medicine has progressed far in understanding the physiology of PMS and has thus been able to better identify and treat this common problem. Approximately 90 percent of women experience some premenstrual symptoms during their menstrual life. Like menopause, it is individualized. The severity of symptoms is broad, ranging from mild cramping to full psychotic breakdowns. The symptoms can be physical, emotional, or a combination of the two. There is no "classic" PMS. There may be certain similarities in symptoms, yet the experience is unique for every woman.

Premenstrual syndrome is defined as a recurrent, predictable, and bothersome group of symptoms that affects you physically and/or mentally. These symptoms can be mild, moderate, or severe; they can be single or multiple. The medical profession is currently debating the semantics of PMS, using such terms as *premenstrual dysphoric disorder* and *premenstrual magnification syndrome*. These distinctions are helpful in clinical research, as they give a consistency and validity to the study of this entity. But for everyday folks, PMS is still the most useful term.

Other Things PMS Might Stand For

- Pack My Stuff
- Perpetual Munching Spree
- Puffy Mid-Section
- Provide Me with Sweets
- Pardon My Sobbing
- Pimples May Surface
- Pass My Sweatpants
- Pass My Shotgun

So how do you distinguish PMS from perimenopause? The first step is understanding that the symptoms, although similar, arise from different sources. In perimenopause, the problems are due to low levels of estrogen and progesterone; the ovaries are functioning less than before. In PMS, the ovaries are still producing adequate estrogen and progesterone, it's just that the balance and coordination of the hormones are disrupted. In fact, there is still a great deal of debate as to the exact cause of PMS, and that is one reason there is no blood test or objective measurement used to make the diagnosis. If you want to impress people at parties, just tell them the etiology of PMS is multifactorial—in other words, caused by many things! To get a bit more technical, PMS is thought to be due to the fluctuations of certain hormone levels whereas menopause (and the symptoms of perimenopause) are due to an absolute decline in hormone levels.

One of the best and most useful methods of diagnosing PMS is a symptom diary. Keeping an accurate, day-by-day account of your feelings and symptoms is the fulcrum on which a correct diagnosis is balanced. There is no shortcut. The secret is the timing and repetitiveness of the problems, and the only way to demonstrate this is by consciously listening to your body and paying attention to the signs and symptoms you are experiencing. It really doesn't take much time, especially if it is a check-off form, but its usefulness is invaluable.

Table 2: Symptom Diary Checklist

Date_____

☐ mood swings
☐ irritability
☐ depression
☐ anxiety
☐ confusion or fuzzy thinking
☐ tearfulness
☐ fatigue
☐ insomnia
☐ changes in libido
☐ overeating
☐ cravings, especially for salty or sweet foods
☐ alcohol intolerance
☐ acne
☐ abdominal and pelvic cramps
☐ bloating
☐ weight gain
☐ headaches
☐ breast swelling and pain
☐ edema (visible swelling, particularly in the hands, feet, and legs)
☐ worsening of chronic conditions like arthritis and ulcers

It is easy for the layperson and the doctor alike to mistake PMS for perimenopause. This is a major source of confusion to many of you who are in your mid- to late forties. Studies have shown that PMS may indeed worsen during this decade of life or even appear for the first time. Some laboratory tests may be helpful in making the distinction. Remember, the lab tests won't diagnose PMS, but they can separate it from perimenopause. There are two hormones that can be measured that are helpful in making the distinction between PMS and perimenopause: FSH (follicle stimulating hormone) and LH (leutinizing hormone). These hormones are secreted by the pituitary gland and are intimately involved in the hormone balance that regulates normal ovulation. When estrogen levels fall, the FSH and LH show a corresponding rise. Why not just measure the estrogen? Because the estrogen is secreted in a somewhat irregular fashion, and a single value may not be accurate. A value drawn in the early morning may differ from a value done in the evening. Also, the range of normal values for estrogen is immense, effectively rendering their usefulness in this instance negligible. The FSH and LH values are much more consistent in their secretion; therefore, they provide a more meaningful set of numbers to analyze.

Simply stated, a high FSH and LH would indicate that you are either in or approaching menopause. There are certain times in the normal menstrual cycle when the LH may be high, so your doctor needs to know where you are in the cycle when your blood is checked. Also, a single value may not always give a clear picture, so occasionally the blood test is repeated and the pattern analyzed.

One of the first caveats taught in medical school is, "Don't treat a number, treat a *person*." That is not to say that these tests are not valuable; they are. But it is just as valuable to know the type and intensity of your individual symptoms. For example, Mrs. Brown may have an FSH of 40 mIU and Mrs. Black may have the exact same value, but their symptoms may be vastly different. This underscores a common theme throughout this book: You are unique, and you can't effectively be helped without exploring your individual circumstances. Numbers are helpful, but what you are experiencing trumps lab work every time.

The blood or saliva tests, placed in the context of your history and symptoms, can greatly aid in making the distinction between PMS and perimenopause, but they are relatively useless out of context. See your doctor if there is any concern on your part as to whether you are dealing with PMS or perimenopause.

There is a great misperception that all women have signs and bothersome symptoms in the years leading up to and beyond menopause. It just doesn't happen that way. As I have stated before, most women have few severe symptoms, whereas others are putting out enough heat to melt an igloo. Nevertheless, the onset of perimenopause is often subtle and in most cases identified only in retrospect. It is only after the fact that many realize, "Hey, all of these things I am experiencing may be related." There is no set age for perimenopause just as there is no set age for menopause. Also, there is no set duration. It may last for six months or five years.

AM I THERE OR WHAT?

How do you know if you are perimenopausal? Start by asking questions. Are your periods regular? Are you experiencing hot flashes? Have you noticed a decreased sex drive? Are you fatigued? Do you have vaginal dryness? In other words, if you are experiencing symptoms of declining ovarian function that are more continual and not episodic, but you are still having periods, you are perimenopausal. Once your periods stop for a year, you may still be having the same symptoms, yet now you fall into the category of menopause. It all hinges on the presence or absence of periods.

What are some of these symptoms? The following table shows a partial list of symptoms that have been attributed to declining ovarian function. Don't let this list depress you; remember, you may not experience any of these symptoms. Realize that God is not punishing you for growing older. A Gallup poll showed that more than 51 percent of perimenopausal/postmenopausal women felt their life was better now (in menopause) than it was before, and a majority of women believed these feelings would continue.[2]

SYMPTOMS

Hair growth	Hot flashes
Low back pain	Vaginal atrophy
Vulvar itching	Vaginal dryness
Bloating	Vaginal burning
Flatulence	Vaginal itching
Indigestion	Vaginal bleeding
Osteoporosis	Painful intercourse
Deep bone ache	Urinary incontinence
Thinning scalp hair	Urinary frequency
Breast tenderness	Urinary urgency
Palpitation	Painful urination
Dizzy spells	Depressed mood
Headaches	Difficulty sleeping
"Crawly skin"	Decreased libido
Vertigo	Fatigue
Vaginal odor	Impaired memory
Night sweats	Problems concentrating
Mood swings	Irritability

It is empowering to become educated about what symptoms are associated with hormonal changes. The trap to avoid is associating *everything* that happens at this time with hormonal changes. Don't wear hormonal blinders! Establishing proper cause and effect between hormones and symptoms is a critical first step in alleviating those symptoms. There is a great deal of crossover in symptoms with other conditions, so be careful not to blame everything on those dastardly hormones.

WHEN WILL IT HAPPEN FOR ME?

Perimenopause is defined by symptoms and represents the months to years that surround the menopause. Remember that menopause is defined as the cessation of periods. The average age for menopause in the United States is fifty-one. Understand that this is a bell curve, so some will cease having periods in their early forties whereas others will see them continue into their fifties. Accordingly, perimenopause will vary depending on when menopause occurs. This time frame is different for every woman. This is also the time when many experience symptoms associated with menopause, such as hot flashes and moodiness; however, not everyone will experience symptoms severe enough to require treatment. Most women will sail through this time unencumbered and unfazed by the shifting winds of change.

Menopause is unique for every woman. You may experience four to five years of perimenopausal changes, whereas your friend Mary may have one hot flash and stop her periods all within one month.

There does seem to be a genetic preprogramming built into the ovaries that instructs them when to begin to decrease their production of hormones. The only thing that has been even remotely associated with predicting when you may enter menopause is the age of your mother's menopause, and even that is a loose association.

There are many factors that may alter this onset. For example, smokers are noted to have an earlier menopause than nonsmokers. Women who have had a hysterectomy (but their ovaries were left in) tend to have an earlier menopause than they normally would, but not by much. Other unusual medical problems such as certain cancer treatments and autoimmune diseases can cause early menopause. Studies indicate that a woman with a higher percentage of body fat (over 40 percent) may have a later onset of menopause and may actually have fewer symptoms.

So the perimenopause is, first and foremost, a time of change that is delineated by the onset of symptoms that are associated with declining hormone levels. It is appropriate to look at the idea of change and how to wrestle with it, because how you deal with change will influence your midlife experience.

A REAL-LIFE SCENARIO

Mary was a CEO of a startup software company. She was forty-five years old, married, and had three children. Mary came in for her yearly Pap smear and physical exam and told this story.

"Things have been really great this year. My company has finally seen some success. Oh, sure, it has been incredibly stressful, but I feel like I am handling it well. I have noticed my periods have become a little more irregular, and I have actually skipped a few. The only thing that really bothers me is these stupid hot flashes. I can be making a presentation to a prospective client, and then all of a sudden, whoosh! I get red-faced and I break out in a sweat. I can only imagine what my client thinks. And I really believe I have lost an account or two because these flashes interrupted my presentation and broke my concentration.

"And that reminds me, I have noticed that I feel a little more forgetful these days. Not anything big, like where I am, but little things like where I put a paper or what I came into the room to get. I guess it's all a part of getting older, which is something I don't like at all!" Mary hesitated, and then continued. "If you get right down to it, what I don't like is this sense of not having complete control over my body and emotions. This is not me. I have always been able to handle about anything that comes along, but now at times I feel less able to do that. Again, none of these things are really traumatic, but they do bother me, and I just am not sure how to deal with them in my life right now. I don't have time for these changes!"

Mary's story is a common one in perimenopause. She has observed some subtle changes in her body and emotions. These changes are not major or life-altering, yet they are noticeable and cause Mary to think about the future. One of the biggest fears you may have in perimenopause is losing control of your body and emotions. You feel like your body is falling apart or you are out of control. These disturbing feelings often prompt you to seek help or advice. Indeed this is a wise approach as they may not go away by themselves.

LEAN ON GOD THROUGH CHANGES

How do you deal with change? When faced with the inevitable changes brought on by aging, do you celebrate them or suffer through them? Do you confront the changes or do you hide from them? Do you say, "I can handle this"? Or do you become an ostrich and bury your head in the sand?

The Bible teaches us how to deal effectively with change. God is unchanging and reliable. In the midst of chaos, confusion, and change, God and his love are constants. Those who have trouble with change are often seeking some form of stability, something solid and unchanging to grab on to to ride out the storm. Psalm 59:9 says, "You are my strength; I wait for you to rescue me, for you, O God, are my fortress."

Those are comforting words when things are exploding all around and inside you, as they sometimes seem to be at this time. Whenever you feel that the world around you is confusing and changing too fast, you can always find refuge in the stability and constancy of God and his Word. Scripture is ageless and is the steady ship in the turbulent seas of perimenopause.

PART OF THE DESIGN

Remember that these changes are *of God*. They don't exist in a vacuum. God does not leave you hanging over the abyss of hot flashes with nowhere to turn. You are never alone.

Perimenopause is a time of change. The first step in dealing with that change is the realization that God is in control and there is a plan for you. But don't fall into the trap of thinking that since God is in control you can sit back, relax, and do nothing. Be an active participant in working through change. You are not God's puppet. Free will and choice imply responsibility. Ignatius Loyola wrote, "Work like everything depends on you, and pray like everything depends on God." This understanding allows you the freedom to face hardships and challenges with the comfort of a firm and unchanging foundation. At the outset, acknowledge that God wants the best for you. You are subject to the natural laws of aging;

however, if you apply the knowledge that God has provided, you can live in the midst of these changes joyously and abundantly.

PRACTICAL WAYS TO HANDLE CHANGE

What are some practical ways to deal more effectively with change? Some of the suggestions that follow may sound simplistic, but your challenge is to actually do what is described, and you will see a difference. Remember, if you keep doing things the same way, you will get the same results. If you are not happy with the result, do something different, no matter how simple. The most obvious suggestions are the ones we most likely ignore, and they can be the most effective. Knowledge is not power: The application of knowledge is power. Good intentions never solved a single problem or relieved a single hot flash.

Here are twelve ideas for handling change. Practice even a few of these simple suggestions daily and you will see results.

> "When we are no longer able to change a situation, we are challenged to change ourselves."
>
> —Viktor Frankl

Balance Work With Play

Schedule time for recreation. That doesn't mean jogging while listening to a tape of the latest stock quotes if you are a stockbroker. That means taking some time to *just be*. We live in a hurry-up culture where it is important to always be accomplishing something. Busyness has become a virtue. That is not healthy. Certainly there is a place for goal setting and industrious behavior, but there is also a place for rest and play. Be quiet, listen, nap, meditate, walk, run, daydream, or vegetate. Heed this prescription: Loaf five minutes, three times a day! Doctor's orders! Often our best decisions and perspectives come while at play. Henry David Thoreau said, "That man is the richest whose pleasures are the cheapest."

Get Adequate Sleep

Get enough sleep and rest. You have been berated with this throughout your life. That's because it is important! Waking and feeling refreshed is an indication that you are getting enough rest. One author recently went so far as to say that if you have to use an alarm clock to wake you every morning, you are not getting enough rest. That may be taking things a bit far. I'm guilty myself. As a physician on call and a parent, I know about sleep deprivation. The problems often mimic those of menopause: poor concentration, forgetfulness, and irritability. On the seventh day God rested, and if it is okay for him, it's okay for you. Make sleep a priority, and get help if it doesn't come naturally. Trying to face midlife and change in a sleep-deprived state is like driving through a heavy fog.

Work Off Tensions

Physical exercise in any form—gardening, walking, cleaning house, working in the yard, or running the Boston Marathon—is an excellent way to work off irritating, angry, or depressed feelings. We will see in chapter 7 that exercise is a scientifically proven antidepressant. God created us to move, and exercise serves many purposes. Don't get your exercise by running your mouth, jumping to conclusions, being hopping mad, laying down the law, or running from the truth! Set a time each day, even if it is for fifteen minutes, to exercise. (While thirty to forty minutes of exercise is ideal for weight control and fat burning, even fifteen minutes can help relieve stress.)

Talk Out Your Troubles

Get things off your chest by talking with a sympathetic friend or family member. The fastest-growing support groups in this country are menopausal women sharing experiences. Talking with others experiencing the same tribulations not only reinforces that you are not crazy but also provides helpful coping strategies. Part of this means being a good listener. Communication works best in a dialogue and not a monologue. There are many well-trained, compassionate professionals (including pastors) who can be of immense help in listening and guiding during this transition. Don't be afraid to bring your worries and concerns to your doctor. It may be God's way of getting you on the path to healing.

Don't forget about prayer. Taking your problems to God should be your first priority. You aren't reminding God of your struggles; he knows them. You are reminding yourself of your dependence on God. Don't forget to listen to his answers.

Get Away From It All

Whether it is for an hour or a weekend, you need that time to regroup and think. A simple change of scenery may allow you enough time from the everyday stresses to gain new perspectives. I know many couples who have a specific date night (my wife and I included). We guard it carefully because we know we need that time to reconnect with each other with no other distractions. It says to both of us, "You are important, and I cherish the time we have alone together."

Some people need time to be truly alone. It is okay to say to a spouse or child, "I need some quiet time so I can be a better me." This is not selfish or aloof behavior, for if you can come back refreshed and rejuvenated, you can be a much better spouse, parent, or friend. This does not mean abandoning your responsibilities and commitments to "find yourself." This is a time (whether for ten minutes or an hour) to reestablish your connection to God and to reaffirm your life's direction.

The Bible is full of examples of people who "got away from it all" and came back full of the Spirit of God. Moses spent a lot of time on a mountain in prayer and meditation. The apostle Paul spent several years of contemplation after his conversion experience before he began his ministry. Jesus went into the garden alone to pray before his arrest and crucifixion.

Avoid Self-Medication

Alcohol is one of the most dangerous medications in times of stress and change. The temptation is to dull the anxiety. The reality is that you need to be at your best, physically and mentally, to positively and permanently handle change. You can't do this if you are loaded! Author Croft Pentz once said, "Many things can be preserved in alcohol, but Christian character is not one of them." This also includes the misuse of prescription medicines, a huge problem in middle-aged women. There certainly are necessary and good reasons for using specific medicines, such as antidepressants. Just be sure to work with a competent physician who can properly diagnose and monitor your condition.

Be Proactive With Your Health

This is a core concept preached throughout this book. Do not wait for an illness to strike before you take action. Prevention is paramount. Studies have shown that people in stressful times or undergoing massive change in their lives are more susceptible to illness. Anticipate this, and take steps to reduce that likelihood by getting proper rest, eating nutritional foods, exercising, and using various herbs, vitamins, and nutritional supplements. Knowing you are at risk for problems allows you to take steps to preempt them instead of simply reacting to them. This applies to handling change. Seek the advice and counsel of others who have dealt with change effectively.

Take One Thing at a Time

Schedule your work so that you can concentrate solely on one thing. Don't waste your time by fretting over how much you have to do. Do something! The key here is focus. Pour your energies into completing one task before you launch into another. The ability to focus on a task is crucial in being able to complete it. Multitasking when encountering change can be a setup for failure.

Change can create a sense of being overwhelmed. Take each problem or situation one at a time, focusing on solving that one task before tackling the next.

Avoid Superwoman Syndrome

This is especially important to women with career and family responsibilities. You can't do everything, and you can't do everything perfectly. Divide duties, delegate responsibilities, and concentrate on what you can do best. This caution is timely because the majority of the households in the United States are now two-income families. The expectations of others (and yourself) can be unrealistic. The choice is one of priorities.

Set life priorities, and then make decisions about work, home, church, and family that align with those priorities. If trying to be Superwoman is getting you down, prioritize. Eliminate those activities and responsibilities that don't fit in your priority list. Streamline, sit back, and simplify. H. Norman Wright says in his book *Simplify Your Life and Get More Out of It*, "We honestly believe that life can no longer be simple. But it can. It's not just an illusion. It's within reach. But this means risking, changing and taking a close look at . . . you!"[3] This simplification cannot be piecemeal, however. It may involve a complete spring cleaning from the inside out!

Do for Others

Serve. Escape from the preoccupation with yourself by lending a helping hand to those in need. We are here to serve, and nothing helps a person effectively handle change better than doing something meaningful for someone else. The best place to find a helping hand is at the end of your own arm. To feel sorry for the needy is not the mark of a Christian—to help them is.

Set Realistic Goals

Goals are important. Most successful people actually have a set of written goals lying around somewhere. A study done of Harvard graduates showed that the people who were most accomplished in their respective fields were those who had written goals.[4] The secret is to at least think about what you want to accomplish. There is nothing wrong with lofty goals, but they do have to be achievable. For example, it would be rather unrealistic for me to set a goal of running a twenty-six mile marathon in two and a half hours. (I can't even ride a bike twenty-six miles in that time.) A much more realistic, yet still challenging, goal would be to run a three-and-a-half-hour marathon. Don't set yourself up for failure by setting unrealistically high goals and expectations.

Some of us may set our goals too low (or not have specific goals at all), so we must be realistic too. There are some things beyond our reach, but not so many as we think. Our goals should be high enough to challenge us, high enough that we climb with care and confidence, but not so high that they are impossible to reach. This is not incompatible with previous suggestions to loaf and take it easy. Goal setting is about efficiency and prioritization, which in turn creates time to chill out!

Make and Use Lists

If you are having trouble concentrating, keep lists and use them. A certain degree of organization is helpful during any transition. Because of the innate chaos of change, having written lists of tasks gives you something concrete to focus on. It is like a lighthouse in the fog, pointing you to a safe harbor. Balance is important here. Don't be obsessive about it and make lists of your lists!

LIFE BALANCE

The stress of perimenopause and other life changes impacts every woman differently. One of the ways to master the physical and psychological challenges of this transition is to be acutely aware of your internal signals. This is a matter of focusing on what you are thinking and feeling and trying to distinguish whether it is hormone related or not. This is where a trained, knowledgeable health-care worker can be invaluable. A helpful technique is to keep a diary of physical and emotional symptoms and discuss them with your doctor. As in PMS, an accurate record of what symptoms are present and how they affect you can be a valuable tool for both you and your doctor. Keeping a written record helps you to understand and identify feelings and how they influence your actions.

I want to introduce you to a term called *life balance*. This is an important concept during change because it forces you to analyze feelings and experiences and discover facets of your life that need balance. Health is

"A recent study of more than 50,000 employees from a variety of manufacturing and service organizations found that 2 out of every 5 employees are dissatisfied with the balance between their work and their personal lives. The lack of balance 'is due to long work hours, changing demographics, more time in the car, the deterioration of boundaries between work and home, and increased work pressure,' says the study's author, Bruce Katcher, president of the Discovery Group."[5]

a state of balance among mind, body, and spirit. Life balance can be applied daily, and it acts as a stabilizing refuge in the hormonal hurricanes.

When you have a balanced life, you are able to give an appropriate amount of time and energy to those things that are important to you. Balance allows women to feel a sense of contentment in meeting the demands of life.

When you are in life balance, you feel it. You are energetic, physically healthy, optimistic, and in control. Others can observe it in your behavior. You are even-tempered, you feel good, and you get along with others. When you can dissipate negative feelings from a stressful day before starting a new day, you are in balance.

When you are out of life balance, others may hint that you are acting out of sorts or seem to be in a perpetual bad mood. Often you feel a vague sense of discomfort, that "I can't pinpoint it but I know something is wrong" feeling. Some specific signs of imbalance are fatigue, vague discontent, sense of helplessness or hopelessness, anxiety or guilt, low self-esteem, inability to make decisions, and difficulty in focusing on a task.

People who are out of balance may abuse their bodies through alcohol, smoking, and doing little or no exercise. They may have low energy and motivation, be impatient and critical, and become annoyed, especially when others place demands on them. Recognize that you are not alone if you experience these problems. In a recent survey of over 25,000 perimenopausal women in the United States, a majority confessed that at times they felt out of control and experienced these symptoms.[6]

You may be asking, "What does all this have to do with menopause?" We talked earlier of all the symptoms of perimenopause. The signs and symptoms of imbalance and the signs and symptoms of menopause are similar. Behavioral medicine recognizes that the mind and body are intimately connected. Being in life balance allows us the freedom to blossom. One approach to achieving balance is through a concept called self-efficacy.

SELF-EFFICACY

Self-efficacy is a belief in your ability to exercise control over specific events in your life. Dr. Albert Bandura at Stanford University Medical School has shown that a strong sense of self-efficacy is the best and most consistent predictor of positive health outcomes in many different situations. In other words, you feel that you can control the event (change) instead of the event (change) controlling you. In reality, what you are controlling is your perception of and reaction to the event.

If you live long enough, you will experience menopause. Those who have a strong sense of self-efficacy believe that they have control over how menopause will be experienced. In most cases, this becomes a self-fulfilling prophecy.

Life responsibilities are time-consuming, and we find ourselves occupied by the many demands of others and ourselves. If your life is to be in balance, you must know what is important to you, not what others think should be important to you. You must know your values, your strengths, your weaknesses, and your goals. Dr. Neil Clark Warren, in his book *Finding Contentment*, states that true contentment now and at any time in life is achieved by being authentic. This is especially true in perimenopause. He states, "You can experience enduring contentment only when you have the courage to be deeply and profoundly your true self, the self you discover when you make careful and solid choices about your life all along the way."[7]

If you believe that you can control those choices, then you will be able to achieve satisfaction in all aspects of your midlife experience.

The greatest benefit of the transition time is that it offers an opportunity to develop a future self, a new balance between output and input. For some women, the decision to balance their lives involves cutting down on work, taking on a new hobby, starting a new job, going back to school, climbing a mountain, or running a marathon. For others it involves changing unhealthy habits, stopping smoking, starting to exercise, and learning what their bodies need to feel good.

The optimistic belief that you are in control, capable, and competent to make changes in your life is important to health. Studies have shown that women who have a positive outlook and feel a sense of control experience fewer adverse symptoms of perimenopause. The more clearly you visualize your ideal self, the more comfortable you will be with becoming that person. Self-efficacy doesn't diminish our dependence on the sovereignty and power of God. It is about choices. As children of God, we are given choices of paths to follow. Self-efficacy is about choosing a path that empowers and permits you to live the meaningful and joyous life that God intends. Know yourself and use that knowledge to honestly prioritize your actions, decisions, and beliefs.

ACTION CHALLENGE

Reread the ways to handle change: Commit to learning and *practicing* three new strategies a week. You will feel remarkably better in a month.

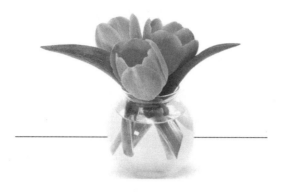

MENOPAUSE: PUBERTY WITH EXPERIENCE

In this culture we are taught from our earliest days that aging is not something to be cherished. Getting older is often demonized and feared. When you hear the word *menopause*, some of you inevitably think old, wrinkles, or Depends. For many, menopause is intimately linked to the misplaced negative connotation of growing old. It doesn't have to be so negative! It is a choice you make.

You may be pining that you have every right to associate menopause with negative feelings. With hot flashes that could power a major city, skin dryer than the Sahara, the sex drive of a coffee mug, and a husband who wants you to "get over it," you have a case for this not being the golden years you dreamed of! It's been said that inside every older person there is a younger person wondering what happened!

If those thoughts imprison you where you don't want to be, then the obvious choice is to change your thoughts. What have you got to lose except your misery? Max Lucado puts it this way:

Life has rawness and wonder. Pursue it. Hunt for it. Don't listen to the whines of those who have settled for a second rate life and want you to do the same. Your goal is not to live long; it is to live.

You think staying inside is safe? Jesus disagrees. "Whoever seeks to save his life will lose it." Reclaim the curiosity of your childhood. Just because you are near the top of the hill doesn't mean you have passed your peak.[1]

This chapter outlines how you must change your attitude toward menopause. The foundation of a healthy approach to midlife is choice. Once you have the knowledge and the mindset, then you can prayerfully consider what is best for you. You are not on the downslope of life; you are just gaining speed!

In the pages of the Old Testament you find a wonderful role model for today's midlife woman. All successful businesspersons champion modeling as one of the most effective methods of achieving success. Why reinvent the wheel? If you can find someone who has accomplished what you desire to achieve, use them as a model and a mentor. This commonly applies to your vocation, but you can also model those who can teach you how to live. One way to change your thinking is to embrace the stories of old that resonate with today. God has provided you with an excellent midlife role model in the person of Naomi.

RUTH AND NAOMI

The short book of Ruth presents one of the greatest role models for the "mature" woman. The details may differ wildly from your life, but the transcendent themes of loyalty, love, devotion, and nurturing speak loudly to you today.

Naomi was a Jew who lived in Bethlehem with her husband, Elimelech, in the time of the judges. They had two sons. A famine hit the area of Bethlehem, and Elimelech decided to move his family to the land of Moab, east of the Dead Sea, in search of more

The author of the book of Ruth is unknown. "Interestingly ... two observations point in the direction of a woman author. First, the story centers on the life journey of two women in desperate straits in a male-dominated society and appears to be from the viewpoint of a woman. Second, Naomi and Ruth's ingenuity and assertiveness propels the story line."[2]

fertile land. Now, Moab was a pagan nation that was the perpetual enemy of Israel, so Naomi and her family became foreigners in a hostile land.

Soon after they arrived, Elimelech died, leaving Naomi a widow with two sons. The sons married two Moabite women, Orpah and Ruth. In contrast to all future comedians' jokes, these women and their mother-in-law got along famously and built strong bonds. Ten years into their life in Moab, the two sons died. It is speculated that these two boys were not healthy, strapping physical specimens, as the sons' names (Mahlon and Kilion) could be translated as "weakness" and "perishing." I can only imagine what was going through Elimelech's mind when he bestowed such loving names on his only sons.

So now Naomi is widowed and without her sons in a strange and sometimes hostile land, yet her daughters-in-law remain devoted to her. In fact, their bond only strengthens. Soon Naomi gets word that the famine in her homeland has ended, so she makes the logical decision to return home. There she hopes to find comfort and support. When she tells her daughters-in-law of her intentions, although she puts them under no obligation, they desire to return with her. With great agony, Naomi encourages them both to stay in their homeland to be with their immediate families. She desperately wants them to find new husbands and begin a new life. Tearfully, Orpah agrees.

However, Ruth steadfastly proclaims her loyalty and commitment to Naomi in this beautiful passage: "Don't ask me to leave you and turn back. Wherever you go, I will go; wherever you live, I will live. Your people will be my people, and your God will be my God. Wherever you die, I will die, and there I will be buried. May the Lord punish me severely if I allow anything but death to separate us!" (Ruth 1:16-17).

There was almost nothing worse than being a widow in the ancient world. Widows were taken advantage of or ignored. They were almost always poverty stricken. God's law, therefore, provided that the nearest relative of the dead husband should care for the widow; but Naomi had no relatives in Moab, and she did not know if any of her relatives were alive in Israel.[3]

Naomi relents, and she and Ruth travel to Bethlehem and arrive just as the harvest is beginning. Naomi knows well the laws of the land, and she tells Ruth that she may go to the fields and glean (or gather up) any leftover grain after the harvesters have passed through the fields. This was a long-established custom spelled out in Leviticus 19:9-10 in order to provide for the poor.

God had made provisions for the poor and widowed. Ruth gleaned in the field of Boaz, a wealthy and respected landowner who was related to Naomi's dead husband, Elimelech. Ruth quickly learns that she has caught the eye of Boaz, a fact not lost on Naomi. As it becomes obvious that Boaz is showing Ruth special favor, Naomi begins formulating a plan to get them together. The months pass, and Ruth is the picture of proper and industrious behavior. She realizes that Boaz favors her, yet, on tutelage from Naomi, she makes no demands on him. Again in a brilliant use of the Levirate law, Naomi decides to put Elimelech's land up for sale. She knows that her dead husband's next of kin is required by law to buy the plot. She instructs Ruth in the proper way of letting Boaz know that she is interested in his affections and waits for her plan to unfold.

There is a hitch, however. Boaz tells Ruth of another man in town who is actually closer in kin to Elimelech, and by law he has the first right of refusal on the land. Boaz, a man used to getting what he wants, tells Ruth not to fret; he will think of something.

The scene then shifts to the city gates, which are like our town hall, where Boaz confronts the relative. He asks if he is prepared to buy the land, and when he says yes, Boaz continues. He states that if the relative buys the land, then he must also marry Ruth. Boaz also states that it would be his duty to father a child so Elimelech's line would not die out. Implied in this, which is not lost on the relative, is that the land he just purchased would go to Ruth's child and would not be passed to his other offspring. So, in essence, he would be buying land that would never really be owned by him. Now remember this is not only about fulfilling the law, but also, and I daresay more important, about economics. The relative is not so concerned about the marriage as he is about losing the land to Ruth's offspring. He ponders all this and finally states that he doesn't think this is a good thing and backs out of the deal.

This was the response that Boaz had counted on, so he immediately calls together the elders of the town and proclaims his intentions to buy the land, marry Ruth, and act as the redeemer for Elimelech's family.

After the marriage, Ruth bears a son who is called Obed, which means "worship." Then, "Naomi took the baby and cuddled him to her breast. And she cared for him as if he were her own. The neighbor women said, 'Now at last Naomi has a son again!'" (Ruth 4:16-17). The story doesn't end there, as we are then told that Obed is the grandfather of the great King David, ancestor of Jesus.

This wonderful story goes far beyond being just an exciting and beautiful narrative. Naomi serves as an important role model for all midlife women. We know Naomi is in perimenopause or perhaps menopause as she states, "Can I still give birth to other sons who could grow up to be your husbands? No, my daughters, return to your parents' homes, for I am too old to marry again" (Ruth 1:11–12). She is past the age of childbearing and so will not remarry.

Naomi illustrates behaviors that are vital for living a healthy, happy, and meaningful life, then and now. The magnificence of the Bible is in its timelessness. Its stories, characters, and wisdom are as applicable today as when they were first recited by the elders around campfires.

MENOPAUSAL ROLES

Naomi's story illustrates three distinctive roles for those in menopause. She acts as a friend, a teacher, and a nurturer—three roles that a woman in midlife is in a unique position to fulfill. These three functions are essential to the perpetuation of wisdom and the bonds that tie generations together. Each of these roles also reinforces the importance of servanthood. Many in midlife, bereft with stresses and strains, would benefit greatly by removing the focus from themselves and instead act for the benefit of others.

Friend

First and foremost, Naomi was a friend to Ruth. She illustrated the importance of friendship between women of different backgrounds and generations. She was family, not by blood, but by bond. This bond was made strong by friendship. You have opportunities to form caring bonds with other women of similar and dissimilar backgrounds. You are bound by your experiences as women and your desire to communicate on a caring level. You are helped through difficult times by God's love and extraordinary devotion to one another. Just as Naomi was bolstered in tragic and extremely difficult times by the love and friendship of Ruth, so you can gain great comfort and joy through your associations with other women of similar experience.

> "One loyal friend is worth ten thousand relatives."
>
> —Euripides, Greek playwright

Support groups, family members, health-care professionals, and friends can all form a network of caring that can help you if you are struggling with menopause. Reach out; seek other women who are experiencing similar problems. Make the effort. Menopausal experiences range from the mundane to the transcendent. Even though each woman's menopausal experience is unique, there is a common thread that ties you all together, a mysterious bond that is shared only by those who have felt and experienced menopause—creating a dialogue among understanding friends. Naomi and Ruth exemplify that this bond can cross generations because friendship is ageless.

If Naomi were around today, I'm sure she would have been a founding member of the Widows From Moab support group! She knew the importance of friendship.

Naomi also illustrates how vital it is to remain faithful to God and his love through tough times. No one could deny that she had known heartache and sorrow. She, like Job, had lost loved ones, stature, and sustenance. She could have easily lamented, "Why me?" and been justified in doing so. However, she models the way God can work through a woman who takes action and chooses to move forward with life. Naomi doesn't wait for things to happen to her; she embraces life and creates opportunities. She knows that God has not and will not abandon her, and he has greater plans for her life.

How many times do we cry out when hard times come, not understanding or trusting in God that there is a greater meaning? Into Naomi's greatest darkness, after the death of her husband and two sons, God delivers Ruth, the beloved daughter-in-law who extends to Naomi her unconditional love. What an incredible support that must have been!

This in turn empowers Naomi to go back into the day and make the rest of her life meaningful and joyous.

God can and will do this for you today through the living Christ. Acknowledge this and accept it as Naomi did. She could have rejected the affection of Ruth and forbidden her to return with her to Bethlehem. This, no doubt, would have led to a lifetime of misery and regret. As a woman in menopause, your present and future years will be infinitely more content if you accept the gift of faith and the belief that God has a plan for you even now. Naomi learned that, even in the middle of great suffering and sadness, God was full of mercy and goodness. Though your midlife experience may not be filled with as many adversities as Naomi (I hope not), the underlying message is the same. Ruth gave Naomi hope and purpose, and with hope comes the ability to weather most storms.

Teacher

The second role that is important in defining a woman's experience in menopause is that of a teacher. Naomi acts as a mentor to Ruth in ways of love, economics, and religion. This idea of an older woman mentoring a younger woman has largely gone adrift in today's transient society. It lies as another casualty in the death of the extended family. No longer do women have immediate access to older family members—sisters, mothers, grandmothers, or mothers-in-law.

Most commonly this situation arises from geographic separation; however, it goes deeper than that. There is often an emotional separation among families that is much wider than any land mass. Lucky and fortunate are you who have a mentor to model wisdom and relay life experiences. And blessed are you who can act as a guide in helping others navigate the treacherous waters of midlife. There is a tremendous benefit to both.

This emotional and geographic separation is a major problem for many entering menopause. You may have no one to consult, collaborate with, or communicate with about menopause. You may find yourself in the all-too-common position of entering into menopause in a fog of misinformation and confusion simply because you had no one to talk to about their experience. You may complain, "My mother never talked about it," or "I was not around much when this was going on, so I don't know what to expect."

God did not design things this way. In the story of Ruth and Naomi, he shows that one way to a proper education about this life event (or any life event) comes not from the streets or books but from caring, knowledgeable, trusted women who have been there and done that! That is not to say that part of your education can't come from additional sources (for example, a well-written informative book), but there is no substitution for mentoring by one who cares about you. Most meaningful relationships are based on giving: giving love, time, attention, knowledge, and advice. The relationship between women in different life roles is also one of giving, and this connection flows in both directions. Both women involved in a mentoring relationship benefit immensely.

Notice that Naomi gives advice on many topics, including love (how to capture Boaz's affections), economics and law (the land purchase deal), and religion (Ruth took Naomi's God as her own). Virtually no important area of these women's lives was off-limits because they were committed to each other's well-being.

I challenge you to seek out women to share in your experience and to discover those who would benefit from your wisdom. They may be right under your nose!

Nurturer

The third role that this narrative illustrates for menopausal women is that of nurturer. To nurture is to stimulate, encourage, challenge, and protect in a loving manner that allows the person to grow.

Naomi actually becomes a live-in grandmother at the end of the story. This is a role that many would cherish but few today get to experience. Again, the separation among families, both physically and emotionally, makes this difficult. We can only speculate on the interaction between Naomi and Obed, her grandson; however, it can be safely stated that Naomi's primary role was that of nurturer.

This role appears to benefit Naomi as much as it does Obed and Ruth. Look at the final few verses of the fourth chapter. "'May [this child] restore your youth and care for you in your old age. For he is the son of your daughter-in-law who loves you and has been better to you than seven sons!' Naomi took the baby and cuddled him to her breast. And she cared for him as if he were her own. The neighbor women said, 'Now at last Naomi has a son again!' And they named him Obed. He became the father of Jesse and the grandfather of David" (4:15-17). So in this role as nurturer, you will not only find purpose but will also reap the benefits of bestowing your care and wisdom on generations to come. It was through Naomi's love and attention that the lineage of Jesus was preserved.

> "The book of Ruth, according to many scholars, was originally part of the book of Judges, but it was later separated. The opening verses explicitly place the book of Ruth in the time of the judges, and it concludes with the Davidic lineage. Therefore, one would suppose that the author wrote the story after the time of King David."[4]

ACTION CHALLENGE

Write down all the roles you have now: mother, grandmother, wife, friend, and so on. Then consider how valuable and unique each role is. Ponder how many people would be impacted if you didn't fill those roles. Understand your uniqueness in God's plan for not only you but the people around you.

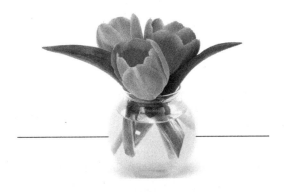

THE FOUR A'S

Let me reiterate what I said at the beginning of this book: **Menopause is not a disease!** I know you may be questioning this after seeing all the potential symptoms and afflictions associated with it, but always keep in mind that this is a normal, natural transition that may be punctuated by various physical or emotional changes.

There is a proven prescription for celebrating menopause. I have worked with, learned from, and helped hundreds of women over the years make this a joyous celebration by practicing some simple techniques. By taking action, you can experience not only symptom improvement but also a deeper understanding of yourself and your body. Along the way, you can forge a closer bond to the Creator, who designed you to be healthy.

The four-step prescription for making this time a joyous celebration is represented by the four A's mentioned in chapter 1: attitude, aptitude, action, and apothecary. These are like the four legs on a chair. They work best if they are all present and working equally. If one is cut short, balance is hard to achieve. Each area is important in its own right, and together the harmony is magical.

ATTITUDE

Attitude is first because it is the foundation on which all else is built. "A relaxed attitude lengthens . . . life; jealousy rots it away" (Proverbs 14:30 TLB). Menopause is the end of periods, not a period of endings.

We are what we believe. Our mindset is so incredibly powerful that it can dictate our reality. God has given us an unbelievably useful brain; if only we would use it more often. Study after study has shown that your perception of menopause markedly affects your experience. A study a few years back compared the symptoms of menopausal women in Japan with those in America. When all the confounding variables were eliminated (including the consumption of soy products), one of the greatest influences on the severity of menopausal symptoms was the belief system of the participants. In other words, the Japanese women, who had a much more positive approach to aging and menopause, had fewer symptoms in all categories. There is not even a word for *hot flash* in the Japanese language! The American women loathed and feared aging, and this had a marked impact on their symptom profile.

What does menopause mean to you on an emotional level? How has it affected your behavior? How do you perceive your own health? These are important questions that you must answer to progress toward health in midlife and beyond. A study done at Harvard Medical School evaluated what factors were most predictive of the death of a person over the ensuing ten years. The results were surprising. It wasn't family history, past history, or even the presence of current health problems. The factor that was most predictive of a person's mortality in the ensuing ten years was their *perception* of their current health status. What was fascinating was that it didn't matter if they were right! In other words, there were people that by most criteria were considered unhealthy; however, if they themselves believed they were healthy individuals, they tended to be alive at the end of ten years. Those who felt they were in poor health,

> "Midlife is about taking stock and taking charge, and the best way to take charge of your future is to have a dream. Dreams give you a sense of direction. They provide a road map for the journey. Recovering an old dream, or forging a new one, can make the middle years the best years of your life."[1]

even if they were healthy, tended to die sooner![2] Our thoughts, feelings, and emotions can have a marked effect on our health and are a crucial part of this balance.

Viewing menopause as a time for growth, freedom, and excitement will unquestionably alter your experience. Margaret Mead, anthropologist and author, described what she called the "postmenopausal zest." It is a cross-cultural infusion of energy that results from a positive picture of menopause. This stems from a realization that life is what we make it and an understanding that God has a plan for all of us, especially as we age. On average, you are going to spend a third of your life in menopause—so it is a time to rethink, regroup, refocus, and rebound!

Charles Swindoll says, "Words can never adequately convey the incredible impact of our attitude toward life. The longer I live, the more convinced I become that life is 10 percent what happens to us and 90 percent how we respond to it." He also says,

> This may shock you, but I believe the single most significant decision I can make on a day-to-day basis is my choice of attitude. It is more important than my past, my education, my bankroll, my successes or failures, fame or pain, what other people think of me or say about me, my circumstances, or my position. Attitude is that "single string" that keeps me going or cripples my progress. It alone fuels my fire or assaults my hope. When my attitudes are right, there's no barrier too high, no valley too deep, no dream too extreme, no challenge too great for me.[3]

Where does this attitude come from? How do you achieve this mindset? You practice! You start slowly, taking one thing at a time, and before long you notice that a transformation has taken place. In other words, identify one destructive belief and work on eliminating or changing it, and then move on to the next. The biggest reason people fail or have trouble starting the process is that they feel overwhelmed. They feel the task is either too frightening or too huge to achieve. By focusing on one negative thought at a time, you can end up altering your entire perspective.

Psychoneuroimmunology

The branch of science that studies how our attitudes affect our immune system is known as psychoneuroimmunology. Multiple studies have shown that how we think, feel, and believe can markedly affect the functioning of even the most basic building block that protects us from disease, the white blood cell. Anger, anxiety, compassion, joy, and many other positive and negative emotions have been noted to alter the ability of white blood cells to ward off infection. Intuitively, scientists have long known that if you are under a great deal of stress, you are more susceptible to illness; now, many acknowledge this alteration of the immune system as the reason why. On a practical level, this means that if you get into an argument with your spouse or boss, not only will you feel bad emotionally, but you are more likely to get a cold!

> "Positive psychology is the scientific study of the strengths and virtues, such as the capacity for love and work, courage, compassion, resilience, creativity, curiosity, integrity, self-knowledge, moderation, self-control, and wisdom... that enable individuals and communities to thrive."[4]

I encourage you to develop an "atypical" attitude. Normal is not necessarily healthy. "Thinking outside of the box" is a favorite corporate buzz phrase, and yet it applies to your beliefs and attitudes. Think aberrantly in the sense of not following the crowd and not accepting what is normal as necessarily synonymous with right. Jesus certainly thought outside the box. He was radical in his ideas and teachings. In fact it was this abnormal thought that proved to be his downfall in the eyes of the Jewish rulers. But it was this same teaching that showed us how God intends us to think.

In the movie *The Poseidon Adventure*, the ocean liner *SS Poseidon* is on the open sea when it hits a huge storm. Lights go out, smoke pours into rooms, and, amid all the confusion, the ship flips over. Because of the air trapped inside the ocean liner, it floats upside down. But in the confusion, the passengers can't figure out what's going on. They scramble to get out, mostly by following the steps to the top deck. The problem is, the top deck is now 100 feet under water. In trying to get to the top of the ship, they drown.

The only survivors are the few who do what doesn't make sense. They do the opposite of what everyone else is doing and climb up into the dark belly of the ship until they reach the hull. Rescuers hear them banging and cut them free.

In life, it's as if God has turned the ship over and the only way for us to find freedom is to choose what doesn't make sense: live our lives by serving, supporting, and sacrificing for others.[5]

Prayer

An effective way to orchestrate an attitude adjustment is through prayer. Prayer can clarify issues, provide strength, and point you toward solutions. Prayer is the mother of all support groups. It is always there, it can be used in any situation, it doesn't require expensive tools, and it works! Ask God for the attitude of gratitude. "May God, who gives this patience and encouragement, help you live in complete harmony with each other, as is fitting for followers of Christ Jesus. Then all of you can join together with one voice, giving praise and glory to God, the Father of our Lord Jesus Christ" (Romans 15:5-6).

> Speaking about prayer and healing, Marilyn J. Schlitz of the California Pacific Medical Center in San Francisco said, "It's one of the most prevalent forms of healing. Open-minded scientists have a responsibility to look into this."[6]

God knows your heart and wants you to follow the path to healing and joy. He can give you the strength. A patient once told me that she needs to ask God to repeatedly give her a checkup from the neck up! You need to ask, seek, and, more important, listen.

God answers prayer in many ways. It may be a booming bass voice from above (unlikely, unless you are Charlton Heston), or it may be a whisper from a good friend. It may come as a magazine article that you just happen to pick up, or from a book you read. It may come in an afternoon talking with your mom about her midlife changes, or simply an intuitive feeling. Use prayer to encourage day-to-day attitude adjustment.

The placebo effect is an interesting study of the influence of attitude on physical health. Virtually every study performed on a new drug employs a placebo (often a sugar pill) to compare its effects with the medication studied. The reason this is necessary is that in every situation, whether it is cancer treatment or infection control, some people get better by just using the placebo. Are they not really sick to begin with? No, it is the power of the mind that heals. The persons taking the placebo believe

"Recent studies published in Proceedings of the National Academy of Sciences using advances in neuroscience (PET scans) have shown that placebos literally reduce pain in humans by changing their chemistry. Researchers at Columbia and Michigan University have shown that the brains of volunteers who believed that what they were taking was pain medication were shown to be spontaneously releasing opioids, or natural pain relief."[7]

they are on the needed medicine, and these thoughts alone create powerful changes in the physical body that heal the affliction. Positive beliefs and attitudes can be effective tools for dissolution of menopausal symptoms. After all, thoughts are simply electrical impulses, and these impulses can actually change your physiology.

Attitude Adjustment

What constitutes a "good" attitude toward menopause? Knowing the following:

1. It is a normal, natural transition.
2. It is the end of reproduction, not of production.
3. Growing old is inevitable; growing up is optional.
4. I can choose; I have options.
5. I am not alone.
6. God has a plan for me.
7. A hot flash is a power surge.
8. I will not suffer from hardening of the attitude.
9. Learned traits of success in midlife include enthusiasm, passion, balance, focus, and togetherness.
10. Menopause is puberty with experience.

APTITUDE

The second "A" in the prescription for midlife success is *aptitude*, the ability to gain knowledge and the willingness to learn what is happening in your body. The limiting factor is usually not ability but willingness.

No one cares more about your body than you. Take time to learn how things function (even if on a superficial level), or you will have difficulty making wise decisions. It is a shame that today people will spend more time shopping for a refrigerator than they will learning about how their body functions. You are handicapped in dealing with menopause without a practical knowledge base.

Not only is it important to learn the basics of how your body functions, but it is also important to learn about your choices. If you are not aware of different treatment options, then you are at the mercy of those who will choose options for you. There are two simple questions you should always ask when you are presented with surgery, medicines, or any treatment plan: "Why?" and "What are my options?" It is important to understand why you are doing something. If you can't explain in one sentence why you are taking a hormone, for example, you need to get that information quickly. Likewise, it is crucial to understand all your options. With any medical decision there are always options. Some of those choices may have consequences that are not pleasant, yet there are still choices. It is common to hear patients say that if they had known more about their choices, they would have made vastly different decisions. Make a concerted effort to acquire this knowledge. There is no short cut. Remember, MD does not stand for "menopause director."

There are incredible resources available today as opposed to fifteen years ago, when it was as hard to find a book on menopause as it was to find a book on compassion at the IRS. Now the shelves are full of good references about every aspect of menopause, and if you Google *menopause* you get over 13 million hits! Educating yourself allows you to take control. It removes the fear.

According to a 1998 Yankelovich poll of more than one thousand women age forty and older, 64 percent can't name the hormones that play key roles in menopause. Forty-four percent say they don't know much about estrogen, and 65 percent say they have little knowledge about progesterone.[8] These numbers are frightening! How can you make informed decisions about your health if you don't know the basics? Educate yourself, go to seminars, read books, and talk to knowledge-able friends and family. It is a matter of priorities.

There was a famous law professor who was teaching his advanced law class one day, and he pulled out a large clear canister and set it on his desk. He then proceeded to bring out some large rocks and place them in the canister, one on top of the other, until they reached the top. When he asked the class if they thought the canister looked full, the class promptly replied that it did. He corrected them and took out some smaller pebbles and poured them into the crevices not taken up by the bigger rocks. He then asked them again if they thought the canister was filled. Again they replied that it was. This time he poured sand into the canister and it filled the even smaller spaces. Finally he asked, "Is it filled?" The class, now catching on, said no. They were right, as he then poured water into the canister, filling it to the brim. At the completion of this exercise he asked what it illustrated. One bright student spoke up and said, "No matter how full your schedule is, you can always fit something else in!" "No, not at all," replied the professor. "This illustrates that if you don't put the big rocks in first, you will never get them in at all." Your health is a big rock. It has to be a priority. Learning about your body allows you to be a partner in its rehabilitation, not a victim of its revolt.

At the same time, be careful, because there is an overabundance of inaccurate, biased information being disseminated about menopause, especially on the Internet. There are many sites masquerading as educational that are really cleverly disguised commercials for the latest fad or product. View everything with a critical eye. In general, if the Web site is selling something, take the information presented with a grain of salt. (See Table 1 in chapter 1 for a list of reputable menopause Web sites.) The application of knowledge is power. Taking the knowledge and measuring it with a moral and ethical yardstick is wisdom.

The biggest health-care crisis in this country today is not AIDS, cancer, or heart disease. It is people not taking responsibility for making healthy lifestyle choices. The place to start is with education. Learning about menopause and how it may affect you removes fear, empowers, and allows you to confidently stride toward feeling, looking, and acting your best.

ACTION

The third component in the four A's is a call to *action*. This has a double meaning. One is obvious: you have to do something to make something else happen. If you are completely satisfied in every aspect of your life—work, relationships, and menopause—then don't change anything. But if you are dissatisfied, to make a change, you have to take action. This is a simple concept, yet it is basic to success in dealing with the changes of menopause. All of the information you glean is worthless unless you apply it. You have to seek wisdom and knowledge and adapt it to your situation. Everyone is different, and what works for cousin Geraldine may not work for you. There is a huge gap between knowing what to do and doing it. Often that gap can become a chasm. It is easy to fall into the trap of inactivity, and there is no greater barrier to success.

The Epistle of James talks about faith without works. "Just as the body is dead without breath, so also faith is dead without good works" (James 2:26). Ideas, knowledge, and faith will die without action. Walt Disney once said, "The way to get started is to quit talking and begin doing."

> "When I stand before God at the end of my life, I would hope that I would not have a single bit of talent left, and could say, 'I used everything you gave me.'"
>
> —Erma Bombeck

If the task of celebrating menopause seems daunting, begin with baby steps. The hardest part of any chore is starting. Begin today by taking the information you have gathered from this book and apply just one of the principles. Next week adopt another; the following week, another. Soon you will be a veritable "Ms. Menopause," spreading the gospel of health and happiness to grouchy old folks worldwide! But you have to start. Edward Young said, "One of these days is none of these days."

Why do people fail to take action? One of the biggest reasons is fear of failure. What if it doesn't work? What if I find out something bad? What if I have to give up something I don't want to? For some it may actually be the fear of success! What if I change and my husband doesn't like it? What if I feel better and have nothing left to complain about? What is fear but *False Expectations Appearing Real*? In other words, the imagination is often much worse than the reality.

Don't let the fear of failure cause you to stagnate. There is only one true failure: the failure of inactivity. Every action begins with an idea, but that idea can die from idleness. The most educated people in the world are impotent unless they apply their knowledge. What good is a guru who spends her entire day "thinking great thoughts"? She may be full of facts and philosophy but lacking in wisdom. Wisdom is taking knowledge and using it to make moral decisions, then acting on those decisions. It is not what we can do, it is what we *will* do that counts.

Benjamin Disraeli said, "Action may not always bring about happiness, but there is no happiness without action."

The Benefits of Action

David knew the power of action. While the whole army of Israel was immobilized, David went after Goliath. With God standing by him, he had no reason to procrastinate. He showed that inactivity could be fatal. The only way to make a difference was to accomplish the impossible. He did!

Jochebed, mother of Moses, didn't stand idly by as Pharaoh's army killed the male Jewish children. She took action, and a nation was led from captivity.

The five daughters of Zelophehad, whose story is told in Numbers, took action and petitioned Moses to grant them their father's inheritance, which would have otherwise been lost to them. Some jurists have declared it the oldest decided case that is still cited as an authority.

Rahab, the harlot of Jericho, took action in hiding the spies of Israel because of her belief in their God, and, for her actions, she and her family were spared when the walls of Jericho came tumbling down.

Esther, Queen of the Persian Empire, took heroic action to prevent the massacre of her race.

Lydia, a successful businesswoman of Philippi, heard the message of Christ from Paul and didn't just embrace the idea; she took action and made her home the first meeting place for Christians in Europe.

Priscilla, a tentmaker with her husband, became one of the most influential women of the early Christian church, not by her grand ideas or her scholarly theology, but by actively teaching her wisdom at Corinth and Ephesus.

These are biblical examples of numerous everyday women and men who took their passionate ideas and beliefs and transformed their lives and the lives of others through action.

The E-Word

The second part of the action prescription involves moving—literally. The dreaded E-word: exercise. God meant for us to be mobile. You were designed to move. If you were meant to sit around all day, you would have been created as a spineless blob of protoplasm. We should be physically active. This is such an important component of success in menopause that I have devoted chapter 8 to exercise and its benefits.

APOTHECARY

The final A in my prescription for success in menopause is *apothecary*. This stands for the many pharmaceuticals and nutraceuticals available to treat the symptoms of menopause. These include prescription medications, such as estrogen and other hormones; herbal products, such as black cohosh; and nutritional supplements, such as vitamin E. There is enough information on this subject to fill the next two chapters, so read on.

ACTION CHALLENGE

Attitude: Tomorrow, jump out of bed. Stand on the end of the bed with your hands raised and scream, "Good morning, Lord!" instead of the routine, "Good Lord, it's morning." It will start your day out right, and the look on your husband's face will be worth the effort!

Aptitude: Learn a new fun fact about your body to share with friends or loved ones. "Hey, Marge, did you know that if you took out my intestines and stretched them lengthwise they would go around this room three times?"

Action: Today walk around the room, tomorrow walk around the block, and the next day walk to the local health club and sign up.

Apothecary: Find something that looks and tastes like tree bark. Eat it. It is probably good for you and, if nothing else, it will keep you regular!

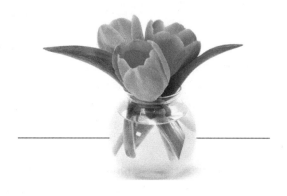

TREATMENT OPTIONS: HORMONES

You are most likely reading this book for one of two reasons. Either you are extremely bright and unbelievably discerning in your choice of reading material, or you are experiencing some symptom or symptoms of menopause you wish to be rid of. Presently there is only one reason you should consider any treatment for menopause, and that is symptoms. Whether prescription medicines or over-the-counter remedies, symptoms dictate usage. Menopause is not a disease, so if it is not broken, don't fix it! For those of you who do have troublesome symptoms, this chapter will outline several options including both traditional hormone therapy and bioidentical hormones.

Hear this loud and clear: Not all of you will experience problems with menopause! You don't need estrogen, herbs, or anything if you are doing well. Don't be fooled by the tidal wave of advertising proclaiming that all menopausal women need something. That is a total myth! There is no law that requires menopause to be a trial by fire (or hot flash). However, for the 70 percent of women who have at least one bothersome symptom, this chapter is for you.

Don't forget that the use of hormones (or anything else) invokes just one of the four "A's": apothecary. To achieve true balance and harmony, attitude, aptitude, and action must be given equal attention. Review the prior chapters if that isn't clear. The use of medications and/or herbs for the relief of menopausal problems is just a part of the solution. Proper nutrition, exercise, and state of mind all play an equal role in celebrating menopause. Medicines and other substances are only adjuncts to lifestyle choices. Medicines, herbs, and vitamins may alleviate particular symptoms, but for a truly transformational experience, all aspects of wellness must be honored. Don't settle for surviving menopause; set a goal to rejoice in menopause!

> One of the earliest known references to menopause is from an Egyptian medical text dated 2000 B.C.: "If a menopausal woman has pain or makes trouble, pound her hard on the jaw."[1]

IS ONE TREATMENT MORE SPIRITUAL?

Traditional and bioidentical hormones are proven, legitimate, and effective options for some women. These are not the only choices, however. There are proven, legitimate, non-hormonal alternatives for virtually every menopausal complaint, and these will be explored in the next chapter. The goal of this chapter is to provide you with workable options and information to facilitate your decision-making process. In all things, you must respect the maxim that all doctors-in-training memorize: First, do no harm.

There is nothing in Scripture that disapproves or forbids the appropriate use of conventional drugs, hormones, or other modern medical triumphs as long as they are utilized in a moral and ethical manner. Furthermore, there is no moral superiority in natural treatments. In other words, you are no less spiritual if you use hormones instead of herbs. There are some in the Christian marketplace that co-opted the term *natural* with the implication that there is some spiritual value in choosing this approach to symptom control over other options. Using natural substances is simply one option and has no moral or ethical implications. I believe that God provides for the needs of all women, and this may take a variety of different routes. Some mistakenly try to debate the theology of medical therapeutics. There is no one approach that takes the spiritual high ground. Unfortunately there are some in the Christian community who have an unfounded disdain for medicines and drugs. They view these substances as polluting the natural state of the body. Not only is this theologically unsound, but it just doesn't make sense. There are some wonderful man-made medications available for a variety of ailments. God certainly works through men and women to provide these medications. Whether prescription medicine or herbs, they are of God. The key is to understand your choices and use the discerning capacities granted to you by God to decide what is best for you. The following pages are meant to stimulate you to explore and ask questions about what will be most effective for *you*.

SAY WHAT YOU MEAN

Before we traverse the turbulent waters of the hormonal high seas, let's be very clear on terminology. You have to understand the jargon to get in the game, so let's take a moment for a hormonal primer.

In this book, traditional hormone therapy includes synthetic (or man-made) substances. In fact, think of treatment options as three separate categories. The first category is synthetic or man-made hormones (Premarin, Provera). The second category is the bioidentical hormones (estradiol, estriol). These differ from synthetics in that they are equivalent to the substances that your body produces and are plant derived. The third category are nutraceuticals (herbs and vitamins). Don't even use the term *natural* because it really has no meaning.

Let's discuss hormone replacement therapy and address when it is appropriate and when it is not. Understand that the following discussion applies to both synthetic and bioidentical hormones.

HORMONE THERAPY

Hormone therapy (HT) involves three hormones: estrogen, progesterone, and testosterone. The ovaries (and other tissues to a small degree) produce all three of these substances. HT should be viewed as a medication. It is not a vitamin, cosmetic, or cure-all. It is a prescription medication (whether synthetic or bioidentical) that should be used for specific reasons. It is unreasonable to suggest that all menopausal women should be on HT. That is like saying all people should take blood pressure medicine just in case they develop hypertension. The antiquated adage of "once you turn fifty, you need to be on hormones" is both wrong and dangerous. The most important questions to ask when investigating HT are *What benefits can it offer me and, conversely, what are the risks?* As with any medication, the benefits have to outweigh the risks. Certain problems make HT much too risky regardless of the benefits (see Table 3). All medications have side effects, and HT is no exception.

In 1930 Ayerst Labs produced its first estrogen product. The product, called Emmenin, was derived from the late-pregnancy urine of Canadian women, and was introduced as the "first orally effective estrogen." It didn't last long as it was expensive to make and had a bad smell and taste![2]

Some may realize substantial symptomatic improvement with HT. Just as all politics is local, so all medication use is individual. There is no blanket statement that is accurate as it applies to menopausal women. In fact, there is a common misperception that HT use is wildly abundant. One study estimated that only 17 percent of eligible perimenopausal women were taking some form of HT.[3] The fact is that those on HT are in the minority! And that is how it should be. But for those it helps, it can be a lifesaver.

TABLE 3: CONTRAINDICATIONS TO ESTROGEN USE

Pregnancy	History of blood clots
Breast cancer	Clotting disorder
Uterine cancer	Acute liver disease
Undiagnosed vaginal bleeding	Chronic liver dysfunction
Active thrombophlebitis	Gallstones

In other words, the use of HT is a personal decision based on your medical needs, current symptoms, past history, family history, and health philosophy. What is right for your sister-in-law may be very wrong for you!

There is basically one legitimate reason for using HT, and that is the short-term relief of symptoms. If you are currently using HT, or are considering using it, identify which benefits exist for you. If you cannot, ask your physician to pinpoint what benefits you are deriving from these drugs. If you can't explain in one sentence why you are taking hormones, you shouldn't go through another day without seeking an answer. It's crucial to understand why you are taking these medications! The key point is that, given the most current scientific data, the decision to use hormones (or anything) should be based solely on the presence of bothersome symptoms. If symptoms are not present, or not bothersome, you don't need to be on anything—period! Osteoporosis will be discussed in great detail later, but let it be said now that using HT solely for the bone benefit is no longer legitimate in most situations. There are other medicines that are more effective in promoting bone health. If you are taking HT only for the bones, talk to your doctor about other options.

Estrogens

There is no single substance available (including herbal and natural products) that, *by itself*, can control as many symptoms *and* provide as many prophylactic benefits as estrogen. Let's look at the types of estrogen available and the benefits and risks of each.

Estrogen exists in primarily three forms in the body: estrone, estradiol, and estriol. The concentrations of each in the bloodstream vary at different times in your life. There are probably about twenty to twenty-five different estrogens in a woman's body; however, most are in very small quantities and have very little effect. Estradiol is the predominant estrogen during the childbearing years, estrone is preponderate in menopause, and estriol is increased during pregnancy.

Wyeth, with $4.4 billion in profits in 2002, increased profits by 95% over 2001, the greatest rate of increase of any drug company in the Fortune 500. Wyeth markets the estrogen replacement therapy Premarin, among other drugs. With profits of 30 cents for every dollar of revenue, Wyeth outperformed the Fortune 500 median by tenfold.[4]

Estrogens are commonly used to treat menopausal symptoms. As previously mentioned, estrogen can be divided into synthetic estrogens (like Premarin) and bioidentical (such as estradiol). Both are prescription, and each has its advantages and disadvantages. The term *hormone therapy* (HT) commonly means both estrogen and progesterone (and even testosterone). This combined use is essential for women who still have a uterus because the use of estrogen alone increases the risk for cancer of the uterus. When combined with progesterone, the risk actually decreases. More on that later. In women who have had a hysterectomy, it is okay to use estrogen by itself. In fact, data now suggests that it is preferable not to use a synthetic progestin if you have had a hysterectomy. (Progestin is a generic name for any substance that acts like progesterone.) There is some evidence that synthetic progestins may increase the adverse effects of HT with respect to heart problems.

For years the controversy has raged on the pros and cons of using progestins in women without a uterus. There are still those who think it is always a good idea to combine progestins whenever estrogen is used; however, the bulk of the medical community feels that this is unnecessary and even potentially harmful. Many of the synthetic progestins blunt the beneficial effect of estrogen on the heart. A large multicentered trial recently suggested that natural progesterone is much less likely to do this.[5]

Immutable Rule #1: If you take estrogen and have a womb, take progesterone to avoid the tomb!

So HT may involve the use of estrogen by itself, estrogen plus progesterone, progesterone by itself, or testosterone plus any of the other regimens. Estrogen therapy (ET) is the use of estrogen alone. As stated, estrogen use by itself should be limited to those women who are minus their uterus.

VARIETY IS THE SPICE OF LIFE

Estrogen can be given in several forms, preparations, and dosages. The most popular way of administering the drug is in pill form. Most people have heard of Premarin, the most-prescribed synthetic estrogen in pill form. This is the grandmother of estrogens and currently the most widely used in the United States. It is a conjugated estrogen, meaning it is a mixture of many different chemical formulations of estrogens. It is derived from the urine of pregnant horses and contains about 48 percent estrone and about 52 percent other estrogens native to the horse. The estrone is converted in the body to estradiol, which is the more potent form. Premarin comes in a variety of strengths and is now available in a single pill that combines it with a synthetic progestin (Provera), called Prempro. I mention these brand names mainly because they are the most widely known, and many women think they are synonymous with all forms of HT. They are the most widely used of the synthetic hormones (remember, the first category of hormones).

There are other options. Another pill is marketed under the trade name Estrace. It is different in that it is plain estradiol, identical to the estrogen in a woman's body. It is micronized, or made into tiny particles, to allow it to be better absorbed from the stomach and intestines. Note that while it is a prescription medicine made by a drug company, Estrace qualifies as bioidentical because it is equivalent to what your body produces (estradiol). The same applies to generic estradiol. Many people get confused because they are led to believe that bioidentical hormones are only available from a compounding pharmacy. (Compounding pharmacies are specialized pharmacies that can actually mix and package a drug on their premises. This differs from most of the large chain pharmacies that only sell prepackaged drugs produced by traditional drug manufacturers. The advantage is that they can personalize a particular hormone combination or dosage, whereas the disadvantage is that they are often more expensive and not covered by many insurance plans.) But both estradiol and progesterone are available in bioidentical forms from traditional pharmacies.

Let me be very clear here. There is nothing magic or special about bioidentical hormones, and they have contraindications and similar risks as synthetics. I personally feel they are better tolerated with fewer side effects, but they still carry the same restrictions. The biggest advantage of using bioidenticals is a greater flexibility in dosing, as we will see. The American College of Obstetricians and Gynecologists states, "Given the lack of well-designed and well-conducted clinical trials of these compounded hormones, ACOG recommends that all of them should be considered to have the same safety issues as those hormone products that are approved by the FDA and may also have additional risks unique to the compounding process."[6]

I have listed some of the currently marketed pills and their hormone makeup in Table 4. This is not an exhaustive list, as new products become available frequently.

TABLE 4: COMMON PRESCRIPTION ORAL ESTROGENS IN THE UNITED STATES[7]

Name	Type of Estrogen
Synthetics	
*Premarin	conjugated estrogen
Cenestin	conjugated estrogen
Enjuvia	conjugated estrogen
+Estratab	esterified estrogens (mainly estrone)
+Menest	esterified estrogens (mainly estrone)
+Orthoest	estropipate (estrone)
Bio-identicals+	
Estrace	estradiol (E2)
Micronized estradiol	estradiol (E2)
Micronized estrone	estrone (E1)
Micronized estriol	estriol (E3)
Combination tablets (synthetic)	
+Estratest	esterified estrogen plus methyltestosterone
*Prempro/Premphase	conjugated estrogens medroxyprogesterone acetate
Activella	estradiol, norethindrone acetate
FemHRT	ethynyl estradiol, norethindrone

*contains horse estrogens
+ plant derived

There are a couple of pills that do have unique characteristics. One pill is a combination of both estrogen and testosterone (Estratest—brand name; Syntest—generic). Testosterone, commonly thought of as the male hormone, is produced by the ovary and is responsible for a variety of actions. The most relevant effects of testosterone for the menopausal woman are an enhancement of libido and a general sense of well-being. It also may help reduce hot flashes in some women. It should be noted that the testosterone in these pills is a synthetic concoction called methyltestosterone, which differs from the bioidentical testosterone in compounded creams and pills.

Combination pills that have both the progestin and estrogen in one tablet are popular today. These medicines were created for two reasons: (1) to make taking HT easier, and (2) to attempt to circumvent one of the most bothersome side effects of HT, the resumption of periods. In the past, the most common regimen for using both estrogen and progestin was to take the estrogen every day and the progestin ten to fourteen days out of the month. On this regimen, the vast majority of women would continue having periods for as long as they were taking the hormones. (Even though they would have periods, it is important to know that they would not ovulate and so would not risk pregnancy.) This means you could be sixty-two-years-old and running to the grocery store at midnight for an emergency maxi-pad purchase. This is not something most sixty-two-year-olds want to do with their evenings!

A wise person (I don't know for sure, but I bet it was a woman) then came up with the idea of using the estrogen and progesterone on a daily basis to still retain the benefits but hopefully eliminate the bleeding. And it worked (some of the time) for some of the women. So a combination pill was developed and has definitely had an impact on prescribing habits.

Don't forget the rule: If you have a uterus and are taking estrogen, then you must be on some form of progestin (preferably the bioidentical progesterone). If you don't have a uterus, estrogen alone or progesterone alone are options.

BIOIDENTICAL PLANT HORMONES

Due to the popularity of bioidentical hormones, I want to elaborate on their use and dispel some common misconceptions. In a wonderful book by Marcus Laux and Christine Conrad called *Natural Woman, Natural Menopause*, these estrogens are referred to as the naturals. This is to separate them from the synthetic forms of estrogen, such as the ethinyl estradiol that is in many birth control pills. This distinction between natural and synthetic is an important one mainly because of the confusion surrounding the term *natural*. Unfortunately this terminology has been confused and misused by many, so I have elected to replace *natural* with *bioidentical*. Let me briefly explain the confusion.

What are "natural" hormones? What you consider natural may be very different from what a manufacturer or your physician calls natural. There is no standard yet as to what that means. Anyone can label a product "natural," and no one regulates or controls what that constitutes. It is the same phenomenon that occurred a few years back with "lite." Foods were called "lite," and it meant nothing until the government stepped in and legislated guidelines for labeling.

A simple and useful definition is that *natural* means it occurs in the body in a normal state of health. An equivalent and more useful term is *bioidentical*. An example is estradiol. It occurs naturally in a woman's body, but the actual substance that you consume as a pill or lather on as a cream is made in a laboratory. It may have a plant as its origin, but in order for it to be utilized by the body, it has to be modified by a manufacturing process. It is indeed the same chemical substance that exists in the body, but it is not just plucked from the soil and ingested. This is in contrast to a substance like Premarin, which is a conjugated estrogen derived from pregnant horses. Nowhere in humans can you find a naturally occurring molecule of Premarin. It is completely synthesized in the lab. Granted, it is partially broken down in your body to various estrogens, yet the chemical itself is a concoction of a multitude of estrogens that are not native to humans. Many women today make decisions about the use of substances based on their labeling as "natural." Natural is good, but it may not always be what you think it is. Clarify in your own mind what constitutes natural, make sure you and your doctor share the same definition, and hold all substances to this standard.

> "In the United States, the market for medicinal herbs is worth more than $3 billion. Many of the plants supplying this industry are [collected from the wild] in vast quantities because techniques to cultivate them on a commercial scale have not been developed.... More than 60 million consumers in the U.S. take herbal remedies. More doctors are recommending herbal medicines, and some health insurance plans offer coverage for alternative health treatments such as herbal remedies."[8]

Estrone, estriol, and estradiol are available as bioidentical, plant-derived pills, patches, capsules, creams, and gels. They require a prescription, and some must be concocted by a compounding pharmacy. Generic estradiol is now readily available at most traditional pharmacies but in limited dosages. Dr. Joel Hargrove of Vanderbilt University has published several studies showing the effectiveness of these formulations in treating symptoms of menopause. The advantage is that they are equivalent to the body's estrogen. They are converted from plant sources in the lab, but the final product is bioidentical, or equivalent to your own estrogen.

Another method of administration of bioidentical estrogen that is gaining in popularity is compounded creams and capsules, in particular, the Tri-est formulation. Jonathan Wright originated the Tri-est formulation about twenty years ago. It is composed of a mixture of estrone, estradiol, and estriol, the same estrogens that predominate in a woman's system. Tri-est *capsules* are available from compounding pharmacies. The bio-availability and absorption of this preparation is somewhat different than the cream, and some women prefer a tablet instead of the cream. The mixture is compounded by a pharmacist in a ratio of eight parts estriol to one part estradiol and one part estrone. The theory behind this mixture is that the estriol protects against some of the harmful effects of the other estrogens. Theoretically, this would make the preparation effective, with fewer side effects and decreased potential for danger. There is shoddy evidence that estriol may have less of a negative effect on the risk for breast cancer than estradiol, but there have been *no* large, well-done studies in women that confirm that estriol has this ability. In fact, the only studies that have shown a beneficial effect of estriol were done in laboratory animals.

Can Tri-est *cream* prevent osteoporosis? There are no large reliable studies that answer yes to that question. There is some evidence from studies in Japan that oral estriol may provide minimal help in preventing bone loss. At this stage of research, it would be foolish to rely on Tri-est or estriol formulations to prevent osteoporosis, especially if you are in a high-risk group. The best approach is to use just the bioidentical estradiol, as it is by far the most active estrogen in alleviating symptoms. Adding estrone and estriol to a mixture adds little except to the cost.

MORE ON SCIENTIFIC STUDIES

It is important to make the distinction between a lower risk of causing a problem and an actual protective effect. There is some data that suggests an association between high levels of estriol and the remission of breast cancer, yet this is far from conclusive. It is a gross distortion to say the present information supports the idea that estriol protects against breast cancer. The information is observational (much being from animal studies), and the relationship between estriol and breast cancer is far from definitive. It is one thing to provide data that shows an association between two events, and quite another to show a true cause-and-effect relationship. It can be said, however, that it appears that estriol is at least less likely to cause side effects than its cousins estradiol and estrone.

You may prefer these compounds, as they are natural in the sense that they are equivalent to your natural estrogen. The Tri-est formulation, with the predominant estrogen being estriol, is not magical in its effects. Like any estrogen use, it has benefits and risks. In reality, the majority of the benefits from Tri-est originate from the estradiol content. Any protective effect from estriol is still theoretical. A physician who prescribes bioidentical hormones can formulate a capsule that contains one or all of the estrogens, progesterone, and/or testosterone in any dose. One important restriction in using a compounding pharmacy is that most insurance companies will not cover medicines made in this way. These formulations work great for some, not for others. You are unique, and so is your response to medicines.

Another unanswered question fueling controversy in the hormone wars is, do the bioidentical compounded creams get into the bloodstream enough to have a beneficial effect on symptoms and bones? Advocates of the creams cite studies that evaluate both blood and salivary estrogen levels and say, "Yes, there is evidence that adequate levels are achieved." And their data supports that. Opponents of compounded cream use state there are multiple studies that show that very little of the hormones actually get into the bloodstream. And their data supports that. (Can't we all just get along?) My guess is that the tremendous variation in these results is largely due to different testing methods, different cream formulations, and the individual variations in women's physiology.

Herein lies a major problem with many of the claims of the bioidentical advocates (and honestly, I am one of those). There have not been, and probably will never be, large studies assessing the benefits and risks of bioidentical hormones. It comes down to economics. Much of the money used to fund large studies comes from either the government or private enterprise (in this case the drug companies). Because anyone can manufacture bioidenticals (they are very much like generic drugs in this sense), no one company stands to reap the rewards of a positive study. The thinking is simple: Why spend millions of dollars researching a drug (bioidentical) when the results (pro or con) will not benefit us financially? There are no economic incentives for big pharmaceuticals to pursue these studies, so they just won't get done. Conservative leaders of national physician organizations skirt the problem by saying that the results of large hormone studies should apply across the board to both synthetic and bioidentical hormones alike. This is misleading and bad science. It is clear that Premarin, for example, is a much different drug than estradiol. Placing all hormones under this umbrella is like saying all monotheists are the same, and we know that Jews, Christians, and Muslims have very different views.

All facets of these, or any scientific studies, should be carefully analyzed. For example, some studies may have only a handful of subjects while others gather data from a larger sample. In general, the larger the sample size, the more valid the study. Patients beware: assessing all of these factors can be complicated. Studies are ongoing about the validity of compounded cream use. For now, we can say that definite symptomatic relief (hot flashes, mood changes, etc.) can be obtained by some with the use of the creams. There is presently no convincing data on the ability of estrogen and progesterone creams to prevent osteoporosis and heart disease. Again I refer back to one of my original themes: God has provided a multitude of options for you, so don't use a cookie-cutter approach. Educate yourself about options and then experiment and see what works best for you.

STICKY STUFF

A transdermal patch, which bypasses the gastrointestinal absorption route, is available that delivers bioidentical estrogen directly to the bloodstream. This is a small adhesive patch about the size of a silver dollar or smaller that is worn on the skin and from which the hormone is slowly released and absorbed. The advantage for some in using the patch is a lack of dependence on the stomach and intestines for getting the drug into your system. This is important for people with gastrointestinal problems or who are taking multiple medications. Also, the absorption directly into the bloodstream allows the drug to bypass the liver, thus reducing some of the negative side effects of the hormone. There are several brand name patches available, and they all work in essentially the same way. The major differences in the patches are their size and stickiness. Some patches contain both estrogen and a progestin. Patches may sometimes stick to the skin poorly or cause allergic reactions; however, they are a good alternative if you don't like pills. Patches are generally changed once or twice a week. There are now patches that contain only estrogen, only testosterone, and a combination of estrogen and progestin.

INJECTIONS AND IMPLANTS

Another mode of delivering estrogen, progesterone, and testosterone into your system is through intramuscular injections. This is a popular method among women who have had a hysterectomy, but it should rarely be used by those who still have a uterus. The uterine bleeding with this method is unpredictable, and the effect on the uterine lining is not well documented.

The injections are administered on a three- to four-week schedule and consist of many different dosages and combinations. The medications are in a medium that allow for its slow release over the entire few weeks. Many women like the injections because of the freedom it affords them in not having to take something every day. Also, the injections are helpful if you can't take medicines by mouth or are on multiple medications that may interfere with the absorption of oral tablets. Injections go straight into the bloodstream and may not have the beneficial effect on blood lipids that the oral hormones do (decreasing the bad cholesterol).

The shots are very effective in treating symptoms and, if used consistently, can help prevent osteoporosis. The biggest drawback to the injections is that you may initially experience a higher-dose release (a rush of medicine). Then, over time (2–3 weeks), the levels of the hormones in your system taper off. For some, this creates a roller coaster effect from the hormones in the bloodstream and is reflected as a seesaw battle of emotions. Most estrogens used in injections are synthetic (estradiol valerate or some variant) and carry all the same risks of estrogen use.

Although not approved by the FDA for this purpose, subdermal implants (pellets) of estrogen and testosterone are available from compounding pharmacies and are widely used, especially in certain parts of the country. They are slid under the skin in a two-minute office procedure utilizing local anesthesia. It is important to note that the FDA has approved the drugs in the pellets (estrogen and testosterone) for use; however, just not in this particular delivery system. This "off-label" usage is quite common and usually comes after years of experience. It's like using Skin-So-Soft as a mosquito repellent. It works well in this capacity, yet that is not what it was designed for. Simply stated, the pellets contain the same estrogen and testosterone as other methods, just packaged differently. Like the injections, these pellets should rarely be used in women who have a uterus. The long-term effect on the endometrium (lining of the uterus) is not known, and the bleeding pattern is unpredictable. Many of the pellets are designed to release their hormones over a four- to six-month period as they dissolve. Studies from Europe have shown consistent and reliable blood levels of hormones from the pellet implants. They are convenient, effective, and expensive.

CREAMS AND GELS

A newer mode of transporting estrogens into your system involves creams and gels. These are applied directly to the skin in pre-measured doses. They have recently been approved by the FDA for the relief of menopausal symptoms, including hot flashes and vaginal dryness. Vaginal creams have been available for years to treat vaginal dryness and painful intercourse; however, it is only recently that the technology of cream and gel absorption has been perfected to allow for reasonable absorption of the hormones through the tough outer layer of epidermis. The vaginal lining cells are much more open to assimilating the hormone cream, and it is only with brilliant chemical tweaking that the external gels and creams gain access to your tissues. There is also an intravaginal silastic ring that releases a steady stream of bioidentical estrogen. These preparations are just another tool in the arsenal of the hot-flash hunter!

NO COOKBOOK

Which is the best approach to HT? Simply stated, there is no best approach. The best way is what works for you and provides the health benefits and symptomatic relief you require. In addition to the overall estrogenic effects they all share, each method has its advantages and disadvantages. Whether it is a pill, patch, pellet, or cream, the choice is yours. It only makes good sense to talk with your doctor about your options. Ask what your doctor would do for a family member. But keep in mind, the decision to use any form of hormones is totally dependent on your symptoms, health issues, and expectations. If you are symptom free, hormones are not warranted. If symptoms are present, then it is a matter of exploring your options with a caring doctor.

There are a variety of ways to evaluate the effectiveness of hormones once you have made the decision to use HT. The best way is how you feel! Use your internal gauge to assess if it is right for you. Often, intuitive feelings and the perception of symptom control are much more valuable than numbers from a blood or saliva test. There are situations where blood or salivary levels are helpful, but in most situations the critical determination is the effect of the medications on symptoms. There is a misperception that salivary or blood levels can guide therapy or tell you what exactly you need. This is absolutely false—no matter what an ex television celebrity says! The range for normal is so broad that you can't use these values to assess if you are on the right amount. A more accurate assessment is whether or not your symptoms improve. There is a place for levels, but not as a magic, singular tool to gauge therapy.

IN SUMMARY

So estrogen can be swallowed, shot in the rear end, implanted in your tum-tum, stuck on your *derrière*, and lathered on your skin. And it comes in a variety of flavors and combinations. There are undeniable benefits to using estrogens. They are very effective in eliminating symptoms, decreasing bone loss and the incidence of fractures, and lowering some types of cholesterol. These benefits are well-documented in many scientific studies, and those who question these particular effects haven't studied the issue and are handcuffed by their own prejudices. Also, there is some evidence that HT *may* have a preventive effect on colon cancer. These findings are preliminary and certainly can't be taken as the gospel truth, but it will be interesting to follow these developments.

There is a tremendous amount of money and effort being thrown into hormone research, and it is estimated that the next few years may produce twenty to thirty new hormone preparations. In addition, it is hoped that many of the risks of estrogen will be accurately elucidated over the next decade. If you are considering some form of treatment now, the best path to symptom resolution is to consider options, evaluate benefits and risks, and consult with a trusted, knowledgeable, and caring physician.

THE DOWNSIDE: THE RISK FOR BREAST CANCER

Every party has a pooper, and every drug has a downside. Don't be mistaken; hormones are drugs. No medication is without side effects, and estrogen, be it estrone, estradiol, estriol, or conjugated estrogens, is no exception. The specter of cancer pervades any discussion of HT. In a recent survey, fear of cancer was the second leading cause both of not ever taking hormones and of stopping them once they are started. A recent Gallup poll of middle-aged women showed that close to 40 percent thought they would eventually die from breast cancer.[9] The reality is that only 4 percent will! This fear of breast cancer has become so pervasive in our society that some at-risk women are demanding prophylactic mastectomies to eliminate their chance of ever battling the dreaded disease.

The scientific community agrees that the use of estrogen alone (without progesterone) increases the risk for cancer of the *uterus*. The debate rages on about the influence of estrogen and breast cancer.

The supporters on both sides of the issue are entrenched and passionate. The reason the general public is confused is because doctors are confused!

Does the use of estrogen promote breast cancer? Is the risk dependent on the type and duration of estrogen use? Can the studies that evaluate the effect of birth control pills on breast cancer be applied to HT?

Let me state assuredly that the answer to all these questions is a resounding: We don't know! How's that for clarity?

The good news is that there are a couple of large, ongoing studies that will finally give some hard answers to these difficult questions. The bad news is that we probably won't have any meaningful data from these for ten or more years. Preliminary data indicates that there is an association between estrogen and progestin use and breast cancer, yet it appears to be relatively small.

To illustrate the dilemma, look at a few of the previous studies on breast cancer and hormones and survey their conclusions. A composite analysis of data from fifty-one studies representing 90 percent of the world literature on the relationship between estrogen use and breast cancer published in the British medical journal *The Lancet* had these conclusions: The annual breast cancer risk increased by 2.8 percent for each year of delayed menopause (after age fifty-three), and the annual breast cancer risk increased by 2.3 percent for each year of ET use. The breast cancer risk after five or more years of ET use was increased by 35 percent. After stopping ET, five or more years are required to return to never-user risk.[10]

A series of papers in which data from many different studies was pooled to make conclusions, called a meta-analysis, again shows inconsistency in their conclusions. Armstrong (1988) showed no effect of ET on breast cancer.[11] A study by Dupont and Page (1991) gave a resounding maybe.[12] Steinberg (1991) showed a 30 percent increase in the incidence of breast cancer after fifteen years of using ET,[13] and Colditz (1993) assessed a "slight" increase after ten years of use.[14]

Case-controlled studies, including the CASH study—Stanford in 1995, Kaufman in 1991, and Palmer in 1991—all concluded that there was no increased risk of breast cancer in postmenopausal estrogen users.[15] What can be said then? Almost all of the studies agree that the short-term use of ET (five years or less) provides minimal to no additional risk for developing breast cancer.

In late 2002, a large study known as the Women's Health Initiative (WHI) released some preliminary data to the press that created quite a furor among the medical community and women considering HT. This study concluded that the risks of using HT (PremPro) outweighed the benefits, and this was reported in the headlines throughout the world. Explosive headlines like, "Estrogen use increases breast cancer 26%," cemented the connection in the minds of people everywhere. It is important to explore this particular study further for two reasons. First, it illustrates how incomplete and biased information can filter into the public forum and be incorrectly treated as definitive fact. Second, it proves that the medical community is still learning about these drugs, and, to their credit, can change their prescribing behaviors based on new information.

The WHI was a blinded, randomized, placebo-controlled study (the gold standard in research) following 16,608 healthy women with a uterus who were taking either PremPro (conjugated estrogen and medroxyprogesterone combined in one pill) or a placebo. In July of 2002, after five years, the National Institutes of Health, who were administering the study, halted one part of the trial concluding that the risks of HT were greater than the measured benefits. In real-world talk, this translated into eight additional breast cancers, eight additional strokes, and seven additional heart attacks per ten thousand women per year. Don't miss those numbers: eight more in ten thousand women.

In addition, they noted six fewer cases of colon cancer and five fewer bone fractures in the same ten thousand women. This means that a woman taking PremPro had less than a tenth of one percent per year increase in her risk of developing breast cancer for every year she used the drug. In other words, ten years of using HT may increase your risk of getting breast cancer 1 percent.

And remember, PremPro was the only drug in this part of the study. This information may not apply to other estrogen/progesterone combinations. It should also be stated that the arm of the study assessing the effect of Premarin (conjugated estrogen) alone showed no increase of breast cancer over those in the control group. This has led investigators to speculate that maybe the synthetic progestin is the bad guy. We know from other studies that the progestin blunts some of the beneficial cardiovascular effects of the estrogen, so this data is not that surprising. This is additional fuel for prescribing estrogen without a progestin in those women who have had a hysterectomy. Also, some large studies indicate that the bioidentical progesterone does not cause the same negative effects as the synthetic progestin. In summary, the WHI study concluded, "Use of HT remains the best proven method to relieve menopause symptoms, particularly hot flashes and night sweats. Each individual woman should understand the risks discussed above in the context of her own discomfort and potential disability from menopausal symptoms. Use of HT is still reasonable for women with bothersome symptoms of menopause, particularly those women under the age of 55."[16]

Does this data change anything? Yes and no. It again indicates that combined estrogen/progesterone therapy should be used predominately for symptom relief. There are non-hormonal medications for osteoporosis prevention, and with the increased risk of heart problems in the first few years of HT use, most doctors now feel that using HT solely for osteoporosis prevention is not warranted. The information is conclusive that if you are at high risk or already have heart disease, you should avoid HT. Most doctors now agree that all forms of HT should be used in the lowest possible dose for the shortest period of time. No longer is hormone use viewed as lifelong. If you choose to use hormones (any kind) to relieve menopausal symptoms, you and your doctor should reevaluate their use every year to decide if you should continue.

Realistically, if you adopt the philosophy of individualization and the use of complementary approaches to menopause, this new study won't change what you are already doing.

So what do you do? It is obvious that there are still no clear answers. Many prominent scientists believe estrogen use has absolutely contributed to the rise in breast cancer. A similar number of people feel it has had minimal effect. Understand your choices. All this data means little to those of you trying to define what is best for your long-term health. If you are afraid of HT, whether it is a justified fear or not, your compliance on an HT regimen will be poor. Therefore, if you have a great concern

Every 3 minutes a woman in the United States is diagnosed with breast cancer. In 2006, an estimated 212,920 new cases of invasive breast cancer were expected to be diagnosed, along with 61,980 new cases of noninvasive breast cancer. And 40,970 women were expected to die in 2006 from this disease.[17]

about HT, specifically as it relates to breast cancer, educate yourself about other options. It is not an all-or-none decision. You do have choices.

KNOW YOUR RISK

With respect to breast cancer, it is extremely important to keep the risks in a proper perspective. There are many factors that must be considered when determining your individual risk for developing breast cancer. Some doctors consider estrogen's role in breast cancer like a fertilizer. It doesn't initiate breast cancer, but if cancer starts, estrogen may accelerate its growth.

Table 5 lists some of the common risk factors for breast cancer. Risk factors can be deceptive in that they may lull you into a false sense of security. If you don't have any of these known risk factors, you cannot be complacent. Seventy percent of women who develop breast cancer have no identifiable risk factor! Eighty percent of women diagnosed with breast cancer have no family history of the disease!

TABLE 5: KNOWN RISK FACTORS FOR BREAST CANCER

Family history (mother or sister)

Early puberty

Late menopause

Delayed childbearing (first child after age 35)

No pregnancies

Age over 60

Prior breast cancer

POTENTIAL RISK FACTORS (UNDER INVESTIGATION)

Obesity

High-fat diet

Alcohol use

Hormone therapy

Your individual risk for breast cancer is a mix between your genetic makeup (family history) and the environment (foods you eat, medicines you take, and things you are exposed to). While you can't change your genes, you can alter other risk factors. Many believe these factors are more important than genetics in determining your risk.

Now, just as jaywalking or playing in traffic can increase your chance of kissing a taxi bumper, so certain behaviors can increase your chances of breast cancer, independent of HT use. For example, being overweight was a greater risk factor for developing breast cancer than using estrogen.

Few breast cancers are caused solely by genetic changes. Genetics are much more important for determining the propensity for cancer to arise when certain environmental conditions are present. This is comparable to all the atmospheric conditions being in place for the formation of a tornado, including wind, temperature, and pressure changes. That propensity exists often, yet only when they combine in a certain fashion does a tornado actually form. So it is with breast cancer. The genetics provide the conditions, and the environment determines whether a cancer will form. There are many other factors that play a role, such as the immune system, so it is safe to say breast cancer is usually not caused by one single element.

Dr. Graham Colditz, author of one of the studies previously cited and an associate professor of medicine at Harvard Medical School, effectively puts risk into terms that are easily understood: "Approximately one additional woman in one thousand per year will get breast cancer while on estrogen compared to women who are not on hormones."[18]

If this level of risk is unacceptable for you, look to the many other choices available.

CAUTIONS

It has been stated earlier that if you have a uterus you should rarely, if ever, use estrogen by itself because of the known risk of cancer of the uterus. When estrogen is coupled with the proper dosage and duration of a progestin, this risk becomes the same as that of the general population. There is no credible evidence that the use of HT increases your risk for cancer of the cervix. However, it is established that the use of HT can make you more susceptible to gall bladder disease; women who have a tendency to form blood clots should not use HT; and since the hormones are broken down and metabolized by the liver, if you have any active liver disease such as hepatitis, you should never use HT.

PROGESTERONE

The second major hormone that is important to include in the discussion of HT is progesterone. Progesterone is the counterbalancing hormone in the normal menstrual cycle. Progesterone is a unique chemical substance that exerts specific actions on certain body cells. Table 6 lists many of the known actions of progesterone.

A *progestin* refers to any substance that has progesterone-like action. It is a generic term for many different drugs, including synthetics like medroxyprogesterone acetate and norethindrone. These are progestins that are commonly used in birth control pills and/or HT. The important point for you is that progesterone (bioidentical) is a distinct substance whereas progestins are a number of different compounds. Progestin is a generic term, and one substance that fits under that umbrella is progesterone.

TABLE 6: ACTIONS OF PROGESTERONE

Provides suitable environment for the nourishment of the developing embryo
Acts as an anti-estrogen on the uterus
Decreases estrogen receptors in the uterus
Binds to androgen receptors
Serves as a building block for other hormones
Blocks estrogen stimulation of breast epithelial cell

The progestins were developed largely to facilitate their oral absorption so they could be effectively given in pill form. Progesterone is poorly absorbed in the digestive tract in its unaltered state. If its chemical structure is slightly altered, it becomes more bio-available and, because it is now a new drug, able to be patented.

However, by altering the structure, you also change its effects on the body. Synthetic progestins have many of the same actions that are seen with bioidentical progesterone, but the synthetic progestins have a plethora of other effects that may make their use less than ideal for many. Bloating, depression, breast tenderness, abdominal cramping, and mood changes all have been associated with synthetic progestins. If you must take a progestin because you are taking estrogen, then bioidentical progesterone, now available in a micronized, easily absorbed tablet form, is your best option.

Progesterone cream has been around for about fifty years and is manufactured in the lab from soybeans or the wild Mexican yam. It is the same chemical (bioidentical) as progesterone in your body except it is manufactured in the lab. The soybean or yam extract contains a chemical called diosgenin, which is converted to the progesterone by a series of chemical reactions. You cannot do this in your body because you lack the proper enzymes to convert diosgenin to progesterone. In other words, don't buy an over-the-counter product that contains only Mexican yam extract or diosgenin because your body cannot convert this to progesterone. You'll be getting an expensive moisturizer, and that is about it. The best thing to do when you go shopping for a true progesterone cream is to look on the package for a list of the ingredients. If it doesn't specifically say, "contains USP progesterone," stay away from it. The cream should not be thought of as a substitute for the oral progesterone, as it usually doesn't achieve adequate blood levels to exert progesterone's protective effects. Scientific data supports the use of the natural progesterone tablets, in this instance, over the cream.

Crinone, a natural progesterone gel, is a prescription drug that is administered vaginally. In England this preparation is used in cyclic hormone replacement therapy and is beginning to be used on a daily basis to counterbalance estrogen, since it has shown good serum levels. In the United States, Crinone progesterone gel is approved for use in cases of amenorrhea, or lack of periods. There are no studies on the effectiveness of Crinone gel in relieving any symptoms of menopause.

Some authors propose that the majority of perimenopausal symptoms are a result of either estrogen dominance or progesterone deficiency. This is only a theory and not well supported by scientific studies. These same folks (many of them laypersons) promote progesterone cream with an almost religious fervor as a cure for whatever ails you. At times, these pronouncements sound much like the "medicine show" salesmen of the

Old West. There is no doubt that natural progesterone cream has a place in the treatment of perimenopausal and menopausal symptoms; however, be skeptical of the purported breadth of miraculous cures.

A recent paper presented at the annual meeting of the American Society of Reproductive Medicine showed progesterone cream to be more effective than a placebo in eliminating hot flashes. This is one of the few good studies examining the cream and its use in menopause. There are many individual testimonials and anecdotal reports of progesterone cream's effectiveness for a variety of uses. When you search the world literature for studies on progesterone cream, you find a scarcity of good scientific work that shows the benefit of the cream when it is compared to a placebo. Often, the proponents of natural progesterone cream cite references to support their claims, but the data they quote are from studies using the pill form. Because these are different delivery systems, it is improper to compare pill results to creams.

Bioidentical progesterone cream is most useful in the treatment of hot flashes and breast tenderness. It is also utilized with some success in PMS. Even the European literature, which is commonly ahead of America in alternative approaches, is remarkably sparse in clinical studies on the cream.

One area under scrutiny is the supposed relationship between progesterone cream and osteoporosis prevention. Some authors, notably the late Dr. John Lee, wrote that natural progesterone cream not only prevents osteoporosis but may even rebuild lost bone. He is the only one to report actual clinical data to support these conclusions, and that data is questionable. The previous paper mentioned that demonstrated a positive influence of cream on hot flashes also stated that there was no effect on bone loss from the cream over the year that the patients were followed. To date there is no credible evidence that states progesterone cream is effective in preventing osteoporosis.

Understand the distinction here. Progesterone, the chemical in your body, can affect bone. The debate is whether the cream form of progesterone gets to your bones in high enough concentrations to actually exert an effect. The current data would suggest it doesn't. You should not rely on progesterone cream as your sole protection against this potentially horrible disease. Also, the cream is not to be used alone to counter the effects of estrogen on the uterus. This is for the same reason: There is no consistent documentation that the cream can find its way to the uterine tissues in a high enough concentration to be protective.

THE BENEFITS

Oral bioidentical progesterone is useful in several situations. First, bioidentical progesterone has, for some, fewer side effects than synthetic products. It is a great alternative when a progestin is indicated for use. It provides all of the protective benefits of its synthetic cousins, and fewer negatives. With the advent of the micronized progesterone tablet—easily absorbed orally—your options have been expanded. If you can't tolerate the synthetic progesterone, you may do well on the bioidentical progesterone. A recent large study indicated that the bioidentical progesterone had a more favorable effect on lowering cholesterol than synthetic progestins and protected the uterus adequately.[19]

Some have advocated the use of progesterone alone for the treatment of menopausal symptoms. It is helpful in some women specifically in eliminating hot flashes, yet estrogen is generally regarded as the gold standard because it is by far the most consistently effective treatment. Progesterone is not a quick fix, but it can be helpful in certain women in select situations.

TABLE 7: COMMONLY AVAILABLE PRESCRIPTION PROGESTINS

Brand name	Contents/Dosage
Amen	medroxyprogesterone acetate 10 mg
Aygestin	norethindrone acetate 5 mg
Cycrin	medroxyprogesterone acetate 2.5 mg, 5 mg, 10 mg
Crinone gel	micronized progesterone 4%, 8%
Depo-provera (injectable)	medroxyprogesterone acetate various dosages
Micronor (birth control)	norethindrone .35 mg
Prometrium	Micronized (bioidentical) progesterone 100 mg, 200 mg
Provera	medroxyprogesterone acetate 2.5 mg, 5 mg, 10 mg

NONPRESCRIPTION PROGESTERONE CREAMS*

Brand name	Manufacturer	Location
Angel care	Angel Care, USA	Atlanta, GA
Edenn	SNM	Norcross, GA
Equillibrium	Equillibrium Lab	Boca Raton, FL
Natural Balance	South Market Services	Atlanta, GA
Phytogest	Karuna Corp.	Novato, CA
Probalance	Springboard	Monterrey, CA
Pro-Gest	Professional &Technical Service	Portland, OR
Serenity	Health and Science	New York, NY
Restored Balance	Thymates, Inc	Atlanta, GA

*not a complete list. All products listed have 400–500 mg/oz.
Progesterone determined by Aeron Lifecycles Lab.

In summary, there are basically three distinct categories of treatment tools for bothersome menopausal symptoms. Remember, not all symptoms demand treatment. The first treatment category is traditional HT (some call it synthetic), such as Premarin; the second is bioidentical hormones (estrogen, progesterone, and testosterone); and the third is nutraceuticals (herbs and vitamins). Each category is unique, and you may benefit from using something from one or all categories. Because of their burgeoning popularity, the nutraceuticals will be addressed in the next chapter.

ACTION CHALLENGE

Answer this question: Why would I consider taking a medicine for menopause? Are my symptoms due to menopause, and do they warrant any treatment? Most important, what are my options?

If you have been on HT for five or more years, discuss stopping these medicines with your doctor. Examine the pros and cons as they apply to your individual situation. Don't stop on your own. Use your resources wisely.

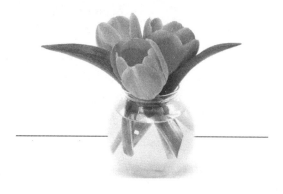

TREATMENT OPTIONS: COMPLEMENTARY APPROACHES

If you are hoping to find a discussion of crystals, chants, and other wacko alternative medicine mumbo jumbo, you'd best look elsewhere. I gravitate toward the term *complementary approaches* because this describes more accurately the non-exclusivity of these regimens. It is not an either/or decision. You can use HT and herbs and vitamins together, or you can use herbs and vitamins exclusively, or hormones by themselves. Life is about choices, and this book is about choices.

Immutable Rule #2: Women rejoice; you have a choice!

Certainly you have the option to do nothing—and for some that is a legitimate choice. But, more important, you have the ability (and soon the knowledge) to look at all the fabulous foods, herbs, and vitamins that God has provided and utilize them to maximize your health.

Herbs and vitamins are just two additional examples of tools God has provided to help you in these transition years.

In specifically applying nutraceutical medicines to menopause, it is helpful to list the different herbs and foodstuffs by the symptoms they address. Keep in mind that your use of these substances, like HT, should be solely dependent on the presence of symptoms. If you are feeling fine, don't think you should be taking something just because you are in menopause. In general, individual herbs and vitamins address specific symptoms; however, where there is overlap, the combined use will be elucidated.

This is by no means a comprehensive list of all possible natural or herbal treatments for menopausal symptoms. You will be bombarded by many anecdotal reports of "miracle plants" (mostly by the manufacturer), so buyer beware! I urge you to hold nutraceuticals to the same scientific standards of efficacy and safety that the pharmaceutical companies are obliged to maintain. The treatments listed here are limited to those that have been scientifically and independently confirmed as effective. The biggest problem women face in choosing complementary therapies is separating the wheat from the chaff. What works and what doesn't? Not all herbal approaches are legitimate, and many of the claims regarding herbal potency are invalid at best and dangerous at worst. This is a highly lucrative business, and con artists emerge when there is money to be made. Remember, *natural* doesn't automatically mean safe or effective. If you are to safely go this route of treatment, you must learn how to utilize nutraceuticals appropriately. Can herbs be effective in treating some menopausal symptoms? You bet they can! But they must be used in the proper amounts, for the appropriate duration, and with excellent quality ingredients.

PHYTOESTROGENS

The phytoestrogens are a category of foods that have such a broad positive effect on menopausal symptoms that they form the foundation of any natural program. Let's start by discussing phytoestrogens in general before looking at specific symptoms.

Phytoestrogens are plant substances that abound in soy products, legumes, flaxseed, whole grains, beans, vegetables, and some fruits. The two main types of phytoestrogens are lignans and isoflavones, two different families of plant-based estrogens. The term is somewhat of a misnomer as they are not estrogens—they only resemble the molecular structure of estrogen, and they are just strong enough to substitute for them in the body. Phytoestrogens are weak estrogen-like substances; however, their ability to express biological activity in the body is similar to estrogens produced by the body.[1]

A study published in the journal *Obstetrics and Gynecology* in 1998 showed that after twelve weeks of ingesting 60 g a day of soy products, 44 percent of 104 women experienced the elimination of their hot flashes.[2] A 1991 study showed that a cup of soybeans a day could increase the vaginal cell maturation, which is an indication of the estrogen effect on the cells lining the vagina.[3] This is important in resolving vaginal dryness and pain during intercourse. In 1995 a *New England Journal of Medicine* article reported that a diet rich in soy (phytoestrogens) could lower total cholesterol, LDL cholesterol (the bad guys), and triglycerides.[4] An article published in the *Annals of Medicine* provided data that suggested that isoflavones and lignans could reduce the incidence of breast, colon, and prostate cancers.[5]

The effect of phytoestrogens on bone has not been well-studied. There is some cross-cultural data looking at the lower incidence of osteoporosis in cultures that consume a great deal of soy and soy products; however, a distinct cause and effect cannot be stated with confidence. Most studies suggest that a lifetime consumption of soy may provide some protection. There is no evidence that an increase in phytoestrogen consumption will increase your risk of uterine or breast cancer.

TABLE 8: PHYTOESTROGEN CONTENT OF COMMON SOY PRODUCTS[6]

Food	Isoflavone content (mcg/g)
Tofu	232
Soy sauce	13
Soy milk	44
Soybean sprouts	368
Soybean, green	1285
Soybean paste	330
Miso paste	642
Soy hot dog	188

PHYTOESTROGEN CONTENT OF COMMON FOODS (MCG/G)	
Flax seed	379
Sesame seed	80
Flax bread	75.4
Multigrain bread	48
Hummus	9.9
Garlic	6.0
Bean sprouts	5.0
Dried apricots	4.4
Alfalfa sprouts	4.4
Dried dates	3.3
Sunflower seed	2.2
Chestnuts	2.1

What is the practical application of all this data? Table 8 lists the phytoestrogen content of some common soy foods. The evidence is compelling that those who suffer from hot flashes and vaginal dryness should first increase dietary intake of these products before resorting to other solutions. You may not need to go any further! If you hate tofu and soy, try various legumes, chickpeas, or whole grains. (See following sidebar.)

Flaxseed oil is a good source of lignans. The best way to utilize flaxseed oil is to add it directly to foods. It shouldn't be used as cooking oil as it is easily destroyed by heat. A great way to utilize flaxseed oil is to substitute it for other oils in making salad dressing. Flaxseed oil is also rich in omega-3 fatty acids, known to have a protective effect on the heart. Most studies report that a tablespoon of the oil a day provides you with the amount of phytoestrogens needed to combat hot flashes. The amount that works for you may vary, and, as with all these remedies, don't expect overnight success.

Another option is direct supplementation with isoflavone tablets. Tablets that contain a minimum of 40 mgs of isoflavones, which is an amount shown to be effective in several studies, are abundant. Most research on these products show their benefits after four or more weeks of use.

Starting your natural regimen by increasing the phytoestrogens in your diet is a sensible approach.

Next, let's look at common individual symptoms of menopause and their effective, scientifically valid, complementary treatments.

Common Phytoestrogen-Containing Foods

- Soybeans and soy products
- Tofu
- Whole grains
- Chickpeas
- Legumes
- Flaxseed
- Cereal bran
- Whole cereals
- Clover sprouts
- Beans
- Tempeh

HOT FLASHES

Hot flashes, surges of energy, heat waves, prickly heat—a rose by any other name is still a rose. One woman told me she discovered the origin of the word *menopause*. She declared it was two Greek words: "meno," which means your skin gets so hot, and "pause," which means it could melt Tupperware! The hot flash is the single most common symptom of menopause. It is estimated that up to 75 percent of women experience this phenomenon to some degree (pun intended). It is important to understand what a hot flash is and conversely, what it isn't. You may be confused by what constitutes a true hormonal hot flash since not all that flashes is hormonal! Typically, it begins suddenly in the upper chest and gallops upward, spreading its warmth to the top of your head. The classic hot flash is often accompanied by perspiring (sweating if you live in the South!) and a perceptible increase in skin temperature. It may occur once a week or a hundred times a day. A hormonal hot flash is not a continual feeling of warmth; if that were the case, it would be a hot flesh! If you are wearing only your underwear when your husband has on a wool sweater, you probably have more of a steady state metabolic variation than the explosive flashing characterized by a hormonal hot flash. (Or you are trying to lure him away from the TV?)

You may ask, "When do I do something about the hot flashes?"

The answer is, "Whenever they bother you!" No one ever died from hot flashes, although many have wished they would. If they are interfering with your normal life, it's time to call in the firemen. The mere presence of hot flashes—or any other symptom—doesn't mandate treatment. It all goes back to how bothersome the symptoms become.

Ways to Keep Your Cool

ℛ Exercise.

ℛ Avoid triggers. For some women, hot flashes are triggered by stress, caffeine, drinking alcohol, eating spicy foods, or drinking or eating something very hot, such as soup.

ℛ Reduce stress. Try deep, slow abdominal breathing, prayer, massage, or a leisurely bath. Researchers have found deep, slow breathing can reduce the effects of hot flashes in half of women, probably by calming the central nervous system.

ℛ Don't get overheated. Dress in layers so you can remove them at the first sign of a flash.

ℛ Drink a glass of cold water or juice at the onset of a flash.

ℛ Use cotton sheets, lingerie, and clothing that allow your skin to breathe.

Alice, a top executive with a local bank, relayed her first experience with a hot flash. She was making a presentation to the bank's board of directors and, at an important sequence in the presentation, she suddenly felt like her head was on fire. She felt as if her twenty-four-hour antiperspirant was on its seventy-second hour! She fought the urge to rip her clothes off (which no doubt would have made an impression on the board). Not only was she spooked by not knowing what was happening, but she also had never before "let them see her sweat." She was a control fanatic, which was why she had risen in the bank hierarchy so fast. But now, for the first time, she felt out of control. She was able to laugh about it when she came and saw me, but only after she was reassured that she could control and possibly eliminate the flashes forever. Here are some treatment options for fanatical flashers.

Vitamin E

Vitamin E has long been used to reduce or eliminate hot flashes. As far back as 1949, studies showed the effectiveness of vitamin E for hot flashes and other menopausal symptoms.[7] The exact mechanism of how it works is unknown, but the fact remains that both the studies and clinical experience supports its use. Most of the scientific data suggests a minimum dosage of 800 units of d-alpha tocopherol (the fancy chemical name of the natural form of vitamin E) or mixed tocopherols daily. Avoid the cheaper dl-alpha-tocopherol (the synthetic vitamin E that is not as proven in its effectiveness). If most of the hot flashes occur at night, as they commonly do, take the vitamin E as a single dose at bedtime. Vitamin E is somewhat better absorbed if taken with food, even better if there is a little fat in the food. (Isn't it great to have something good to say about fat?!) Vitamin E is a fat-soluble vitamin, meaning it has the potential to be stored in the fat cells of the body; however, dosages of up to 2,000 international units (IU) a day have been shown to be safe. Vitamin E can be found in vegetable oils, almonds, walnuts, margarine, spinach, lettuce, and onions.

Vitamin E is also associated with a variety of other health benefits. It is a powerful antioxidant and has been shown to decrease the incidence of heart disease in certain individuals. It may protect from some types of cancers. You should avoid vitamin E if you are on any blood thinners or anticipate surgery in the next few weeks, as this vitamin has been associated with interfering with the blood clotting mechanism. Most multivitamin preparations contain only a smidge of vitamin E, so if you want to extinguish the flashes, you probably will need to supplement the vitamin E separately.

Black Cohosh

Cimicifuga racemosa, or black cohosh, is one of the most studied and utilized herbs for the elimination of hot flashes. Black cohosh is a beautiful long, drooping raceme with delicate white flowers and is native to the United States. The medicinal part of the plant is the dried root. This herb has been used by Native Americans for centuries for a variety of female complaints.

Remifemin is a proprietary product that contains a standardized dose of triterpenes, one of the active ingredients of black cohosh. This particular product has been widely used in Germany for years and has valid studies that support its effectiveness and safety. An article in the *Journal of Women's Health* concludes that Cimicifuga racemosa is extremely effective in treating hot flashes and other menopausal symptoms.[8]

Several randomized, double-blind, placebo-controlled studies have demonstrated the effectiveness of Remifemin on hot flashes, vaginal dryness, and mood changes. One of the most interesting and telling studies was published in 1988. It compared Remifemin with estriol and Premarin, and tested their effects on controlling various menopausal symptoms. This study used the Kupperman Menopausal Scale, a long-validated measure of symptom intensity. The results showed that there was no significant difference among any of the treatment groups, and *all* were effective in reducing the frequency and intensity of symptoms.[9] A study done a few years earlier compared Remifemin with Premarin .625 mg and Valium 2 mg in the treatment of hot flashes. Remifemin was found to be superior to both![10]

The data indicates that the most appropriate beginning dose is one tablet twice a day (20 mg per tablet). If you have not seen significant improvement by the first month, increase the dosage to two tablets twice a day. The safety of black cohosh is exceptional and has been studied and documented in over sixty years of use in Germany.[11] Remifemin Plus is a new product containing black cohosh and Saint-John's-wort, which will be discussed in the section on moods.

I mention this brand name to highlight a problem with the herbal medicine industry as a whole. There is virtually no government regulation of these products and often what appears on the label is not exactly what you get in the bottle. Going to the pharmacy and picking up a bottle of "generic" black cohosh (or any herb) is a little like playing the lottery. You hope you get a winner, but odds are against you. That is why it is critical that you become familiar with a few reputable manufacturers—many of which I list in this chapter—and seek out their products. Remember, garbage in equals garbage out. Be a critical consumer.

Progesterone Cream

As I mentioned in chapter 6, there is evidence that bioidentical progesterone cream is helpful for many menopausal symptoms. It is most useful in addition to other treatments for hot flashes. Two papers at the 2002 meeting of the World Congress on Fertility and Sterility showed significant improvement in hot flashes for women using progesterone cream versus a placebo cream.[12] There are many anecdotal reports of its effectiveness, and more investigations will be forthcoming. The cream can be obtained over the counter or in compounding pharmacies with a prescription. Use $^1/_4$–$^1/_2$ teaspoon (about 30 mg) twice a day rubbed on the abdomen, buttocks, or breast. Progesterone cream is used for a variety of ailments, including PMS, but at different dosing amounts and frequency.

If you use the over-the-counter progesterone cream, make sure that it actually contains progesterone. Many advertised as "wild yam cream" or "natural progesterone" actually contain the precursor of progesterone and not the actual hormone. Your body cannot convert these precursor substances to progesterone, so these creams are basically expensive moisturizers. If the contents label doesn't actually say "contains USP progesterone," leave it alone. You may have a tough time finding content labels on some products, as they are so shoddy they don't want you to know what is in them. Needless to say, these products are about as useful as a screen door on a submarine! As with many herbal and natural solutions, it is largely a trial-and-error approach since the absorption of the cream varies in different women. Refer back to chapter 6 for a list of brand name progesterone creams that have been independently tested.

Other Approaches

Although they are not treatments in the true sense of the word, two dietary restrictions are important in reducing and eliminating hot flashes. Sometimes it is more important to eliminate aggravating factors than to treat existing symptoms. You may not be aware that you are exacerbating your problems by doing certain things.

First, get rid of caffeine in your life! This powerful drug can ignite hot flashes with a passion. Eliminating or reducing sodas, coffee, tea, and chocolate will help in most cases. And don't forget those caffeine-containing headache remedies.

Eliminating alcohol can also reduce hot flashes. Alcohol—red wine in particular—has been identified as a trigger for the flashes. You booze, you lose!

Stress has also been shown to be a major inducer of hot flashes. Even if the hot flashes are presently controlled, you may see an exacerbation of the power surges during high-stress situations.

Several herbs have been touted as fire extinguishers for hot flashes, including dong quai, borage seed oil, licorice root, and motherwort leaf. But these remedies suffer the same problem as many herbal preparations—most of the information is anecdotal. Use proven remedies first before choosing these herbs. If the established approaches are unsuccessful, then it would be worthwhile to experiment with these second-line substances.

In resistant cases, where nothing else works (including estrogen), medicines commonly used as antidepressants (Zoloft, Effexor, etc.) can be prescribed. These substances are thought to dampen hot flashes by their effect on serotonin, a brain hormone. They are particularly helpful if you have any of the problems that prohibit the use of estrogen, such as breast cancer or blood clots. Other non-hormonal prescription medicines that have been used for hot flashes include Neurontin, Bellergal, and Megace.

Treatment Summary for Hot Flashes

1. Minimize stress.
2. Increase phytoestrogens in your diet or use isoflavone supplements.
3. Decrease caffeine and alcohol.
4. Exercise.
5. Take vitamin E (800 units a day minimum).
6. Try Remifemin (black cohosh), one to two tablets twice a day.
7. Use a quality progesterone cream ($^1/_4$–$^1/_2$ teaspoon twice a day).
8. Try bioidentical estrogen tablets or cream.
9. Try a non-hormonal prescription medicine.

Follow a step-by-step approach. Start with number one and work your way down. *Everyone* can reduce or eliminate hot flashes through one or a combination of these tools.

MOOD CHANGES AND MILD DEPRESSION

Many of you know from experience that there is a link between menopause and moods. This becomes most apparent as you yell at your kids for looking at you the wrong way. Next to hot flashes, surveys show that an alteration in mood is the most common symptom of menopause.

There is a link between estrogen and serotonin, an important brain hormone that has a marked effect on moods and emotions. This may be why you can see behavioral changes during times of estrogen variation, such as puberty, postpartum, and menopause. Estrogen can act as a modulator in the metabolism of this hormone, and that in turn alters emotions. The lack of estrogen has a bearing on how serotonin is processed by the body. There is mounting evidence that the brain actually contains receptors that snatch estrogen out of the bloodstream. The research seems to indicate that hormones influence brain chemistry to a greater degree than once thought.

Don't despair; you may never experience mood changes in menopause, or you may experience subtle, temporary alterations that only you notice. It is good to be sensitive to these changes, yet they may be of such minimal consequence that they rarely warrant much intervention. The regimens discussed here are most useful if you notice a disruption of normal functioning, a change in your ability to enjoy life, or a breakdown in interpersonal relationships.

A word of caution: There are many things that can elicit such changes. Midlife is a normally stressful time. Career changes, kids leaving, kids coming back, spouses retiring—all these can impact your emotional dance through midlife. Your biggest mistake is automatically attributing all your emotional changes to hormones. Doctors are notorious for perpetuating this myth because it is much easier to treat you with a pill than to listen to you talk about your broken marriage or troublesome kids. Women are often quite adept at denial regarding their emotional health. "I didn't do anything about it because I thought it was just hormones." "I'm not depressed; my hormones are just out of balance." "Yes, my husband is having an affair, but if I could just get back on track with these hormones, things would work out!" Don't wear hormone blinders. Certainly menopausal changes can elicit emotional upheavals; use this time to take an honest look at your stress level, your relationships, your job, physical problems, or medications you may be taking. They all can have a marked effect on your emotions and behavior. The hormonal changes of menopause often act as modulators of underlying stress and anxiety: they intensify the experience and your response to it.

"Depressive disorders affect approximately 18.8 million American adults, or about 9.5% of the U.S. population age 18 and older, in a given year. This includes major depressive disorder, dysthymic disorder, and bipolar disorder."[13]

Melinda's Story

Melinda called me late one night. "Doc, I'm on an emotional roller coaster. One minute I'm up, the next I'm down. My boss says I'd better get straightened out or I may be out of a job." Melinda is fifty-two, the mother of two high school students, and a full-time secretary at a local law firm. Her story is a common one. She was concerned about the mood changes that she had begun to notice about two years ago. Her initial thoughts were, *No big deal. It's just hormones. It will pass.*

She began taking bioidentical estrogen about a year ago and noticed that the moods seemed to level out. But over the past six months her sleep was becoming more disrupted and her stress level was climbing. Her job was placing more demands on her; the workload had increased dramatically, while the number of people doing the work stayed the same. Her kids were, well, just teenagers. She described herself as "a rubber band wound tight." She really had no other complaints other than "stuff in my head."

Melinda was experiencing many of the symptoms of overload, and the key to her feeling better was distinguishing between what was hormones and what was stress. This is often a difficult distinction. For Melinda, it turned out that it was a combination of both—as it often is. In her case, it was critical to address the hormonal changes along with a referral to a good counselor. I changed her hormone dose, and two months later she was actively practicing several stress-management techniques and feeling much less burdened.

HT can have a mood-elevating effect because of the serotonin-estrogen interaction. I vividly remember a vivacious, middle-aged woman who came into my office one month after I placed her on estradiol. She gave me a gorgeous painting she had recently completed. She said it had been a year since she had felt like painting, and she didn't know why. She felt that creative spark again soon after starting on the medicine, and her low mood lifted. So in proper context and for the right reasons, HT can be beneficial. But it's not always about medicines. Keep in mind that you have options. Here are a few.

Black Cohosh

Once again, our friend black cohosh has been shown in studies to improve mood and treat depressive symptoms secondary to menopause. A study in 1964 had 135 patients using Remifemin, one tablet twice a day, exhibit significant improvement in moods as measured over a two-month period. Another work published in 1987 showed a significant reduction on the Hamilton Anxiety Scale in black cohosh users as compared to a placebo.[14] Most herbs like black cohosh will take from three to six weeks to show any benefit. The key to success is consistency, persistence, and good quality and quantity of herbs. Just recently the manufacturer has come out with Remifemin Plus, which contains black cohosh and Saint-John's-wort. This herbal combination is most helpful in mild instances of moodiness and depression. Let me reiterate at this point that these herbs should be tried only in cases of mild depression. They have not been shown to be helpful in more severe situations. If you are not sure where you fall, consult your doctor.

Exercise

It's been proven that moderate exercise has undeniable mental and physical benefits. This should be an integral component of anyone's "feel good" prescription. Walking, swimming, aerobics—anything to get your heart rate elevated for thirty to forty minutes three times a week is good. At this level, more is better. You won't overdose on exercise.

God's creation is so miraculous that doing something that will improve our physical health helps us mentally. Covert Bailey, author and exercise expert, says, "Adaptation to exercise also produces a mental adaptation. Highly fit people usually have three personality traits: They perform well in stress/challenge tests, they exhibit emotional stability, and they are more resistant to depression and anxiety."[15] There are also many well-recognized psychological benefits of exercise. A fascinating study published in the *Archives of Internal Medicine* in 1999 compared the effect of exercise and Zoloft, a much prescribed antidepressant, on mild depression. The authors concluded, "An exercise training program may be considered an alternative to antidepressants for treatment of depression in older persons. Although antidepressants may facilitate a more rapid initial therapeutic response than exercise, after 16 weeks of treatment exercise was equally effective in reducing depression among patients with mild depression."[16]

5HTP

5-Hydroxytryptophan (5HTP) is an amino acid produced by the body that is important as a building block of the neurohormone serotonin. It is also found in Griffonia simplicifolia, a plant found in West Africa. (I suspect we are going to hear a lot more in the ensuing years about serotonin and its impact on emotions.) In a study published in *Psychopathology* in 1991, 5HTP was shown to be equal to Fluvoxamine, a prescription antidepressant, in treating mild depression.[17] The patients received 100 mg of 5HTP three times a day for six weeks. The 5HTP group also reported a quicker onset of action than the Fluvoxamine patients. The side effect profile was of major importance. Patient satisfaction was higher with 5HTP, and it was better tolerated. 5HTP can be found in most health food stores and from reliable nutraceutical companies. In recent years this substance has been more difficult to find, as there was an episode of a contaminated batch from one manufacturer, effectively removing it from the shelves for a while. Always tell your doctor if you are using this or any herb, as there can be interactions with other medicines. Don't ever stop a prescribed medicine and substitute an herbal medicine without discussing it with your physician. Like prescription medicines, herbal medicines don't work for everyone, and their success or failure often depends on dosage and quality.

Saint-John's-Wort

The winner of the "I am not going to take that because of its weird name" award is Saint-John's-wort (Hypericum perforatum). This herb has received much attention from the press and others. As is often the case with the media, the "facts" are often incomplete or misleading. The standardized extract of Hypericum (3 percent) is the most studied and scrutinized of any treatments of mood disorders in the complementary arsenal. In a summary of nine different studies, Saint-John's-wort showed a decrease in depression symptoms in 59 percent of patients as compared to 20 percent in placebo use.[18] A 1994 study by Vorbach compared Saint-John's-wort to Imipramine, a well-known prescription antidepressant. Of sixty-seven patients using Saint-John's-wort, forty-two showed a positive response, whereas with the sixty-eight patients using the Imipramine, thirty-seven showed a positive response. Saint-John's-wort was reported to have fewer side effects and better patient tolerance and acceptability.[19]

An excellent review article in 1996 looked at all the scientifically sound studies done with Saint-John's-wort. The authors concluded from all the data that Hypericum extracts were more effective than a placebo in the treatment of mild to moderate depression.[20] One notable side effect is increased photosensitivity (tendency to sunburn). Discontinue the herb at least two weeks before a beach vacation or, better yet, stay out of the midday rays.

This is not a quick fix. The average time for the onset of action for this herb is four to six weeks. However, studies confirm that persistence and consistency pay off. This is not for people who are severely depressed or suicidal. All of the studies listed here report some effectiveness for mild to moderate depression. If you or someone you know is very depressed and is a potential danger to themselves or others, seek immediate help. Don't experiment with herbs in this scenario. Realistically, not everyone will see an improvement on herbal medicines, so don't neglect other options if you are not feeling better after an adequate trial.

A generally accepted dose for effectiveness is 300 mg of 3 percent hypericin three times a day. Don't be misled; this is not effective as a quick fix to just "feel better." This is meant to be a long-term approach to a mild problem. Serious depression is rarely alleviated by this herb, and it should not be used in this scenario. Don't hesitate to consult a counselor, doctor, or pastor if you feel your depression is severe. This herb should not be used in conjunction with other antidepressant medicines. Remember that the most effective treatment for depression combines counseling and introspection along with a correction of the neurohormonal imbalance.

Ginkgo Biloba

Ginkgo is the oldest-living tree species in the world. For women over fifty, Ginkgo biloba has been shown to be effective in reducing scores on the Hamilton Depression Scale, a measure of depressive feelings.[21] Interestingly, these same investigators found that Ginkgo biloba improved the effect of standard antidepressants when used together. Ginkgo has long been touted a memory enhancer; however, most of the clinical work shows that this benefit may be limited to people over fifty. No one has been able to explain why this is specific to this age group. Animal studies suggest the mechanism of action revolves around the increase in serotonin receptors by Ginkgo.

Ginkgo is also known to increase blood flow in small vessels, thereby improving the symptoms of decreased blood flow to the brain, such as poor memory and confusion. A randomized, double-blind, placebo-controlled study published in the *Journal of the American Medical Association* reported that Ginkgo biloba extract may slow the progression of Alzheimer's disease.[22] A typical dose found to be effective is 80 mg three times a day (standardized extract). It can be combined with other herbs such as Saint-John's-wort. The proposed mechanism of action of Ginkgo would actually be synergistic and may enhance the action of both. Ginkgo may interfere with blood clotting, so it should be stopped before any surgery and should never be combined with other blood-thinning medications such as aspirin or Coumadin.

Treatment Summary for Mood Changes and Mild Depression

1. Pray, immerse yourself in the Word, and ask God for guidance. (Not bad advice for any problems you have!)

2. Exercise, three times a week for thirty to forty minutes (ideally every day).

3. Try Saint-John's-wort (300 mg three times a day). Don't take if you are already on an antidepressant.

4. Take 5HTP (100 mg three times a day).

5. If over fifty, take Ginkgo biloba (80 mg three times a day).

6. Talk to a Christian counselor.

7. Some may benefit from traditional antidepressant treatment; don't rule it out!

8. Do something! The biggest mistake is thinking you will snap out of it.

STRESS AND ANXIETY

Menopause and perimenopause are ripe with stress. Change is stressful by itself, but magnify this with social and environmental stresses and this time is a perfect setup for anxiety. Studies report that up to 70 percent of physician office visits are anxiety related. Stress is pervasive throughout society. I get stressed just thinking and writing about all the stress!

Hans Selye, noted psychologist and pioneer in the field of stress research, defined stress as the nonspecific response of the organism to any pressure or demand. The operative phrase in this definition is "nonspecific response." It is the perception of the person that defines a stress or stressor. Dr. Martin Seligman, who has done extensive research on optimism and health, writes that it is not the potential stressor itself but how it is perceived that is important. He goes on to say that how you handle the pressure or demand will determine whether or not it will lead to stress. The million-dollar question is, how do you reduce stress in your life? What can you do, beginning today, that can have an impact on lowering your stress level? You can't eliminate stress. What you desire is an effective way of reducing it and dealing with what remains. You will never be stress free; no one is, especially in midlife.

Introspection is an absolutely vital step, because the road to effective management of stress is only successfully traveled by correctly identifying its source. That way you don't fall into the trap of simply treating symptoms and not causes. Treating symptoms is like a dog chasing his tail: You usually get nowhere and end up mad! Inevitably, it is only a temporary fix and can often even contribute to the problem.

> Seventy-five percent of the general population experiences at least some stress every two weeks. Half of those experience moderate or high levels of stress during the same two-week period.[23]

Effective stress management is a twofold process. First, identify the stressor and its source. Second, confront it. This is a healthy approach and certainly one that will endure beyond the short term. There are certain situations in which some medications are justified, but only on a short-term basis and only to get you to a point mentally that you can begin the real work of stress relief. Anti-anxiety medications can be helpful, but always remember they are treating a symptom and not a cause. They are like a psychic Band-Aid, not a permanent solution.

I am convinced that a needed addition to any treatment for anxiety is prayer and a deep understanding that God is with you and will see you through any problem or hardship. Often God works through others in dispelling anxiety. Of course, you have to be open and accepting of that grace.

An effective tool for stress management is to stop focusing on your own problems and help someone else. This is a powerful way of shifting the emphasis from "Woe is me" to "Whoa, it's me!" Perhaps the most illuminating advice on worry and anxiety comes from Matthew's gospel. Jesus is talking to the people about many subjects, and he speaks directly to you and me when he says:

> That is why I tell you not to worry about everyday life—whether you have enough food and drink, or enough clothes to wear. Isn't life more than food, and your body more than clothing? Look at the birds. They don't plant or harvest or store food in barns, for your heavenly Father feeds them. And aren't you far more valuable to him than they are? Can all your worries add a single moment to your life?
>
> And why worry about your clothing? Look at the lilies of the field and how they grow. They don't work or make their clothing, yet Solomon in all his glory was not dressed as beautifully as they are. And if God cares so wonderfully for wildflowers that are here today and thrown into the fire tomorrow, he will certainly care for you. Why do you have so little faith?
>
> So don't worry about these things, saying, "What will we eat? What will we drink? What will we wear?" These things dominate the thoughts of unbelievers, but your heavenly Father already knows all your needs. Seek the Kingdom of God above all else, and live righteously, and he will give you everything you need.
>
> So don't worry about tomorrow, for tomorrow will bring its own worries. Today's trouble is enough for today. (6:25–34)

This message should be shouted from the windows of Wall Street to the palm trees of Pasadena. It is the ultimate hope for this anxiety-ridden world. God provides solutions for our troubles through prayer, friends, family, fellowship, church, counseling, medicines, and nutraceuticals. Don't miss the message here: These tools are acceptable to use in helping with depression or stress; they are of God. It is just as important to realize that they are only part of the picture. All the various tools can be utilized to achieve balance in mind, body, and spirit.

Two herbs that have been used for anxiety are Valerian (Valeriana officinalis) and Kava (Piper methysticum). Valerian, a bright pink-and-white-flowered rhizome native to Europe, is thought to exert its sedating effect by stimulating the release of GABA, a brain neurotransmitter.[24] It is mainly used for sleep, but its calming effect is helpful in chronic anxiety.

Kava is a plant indigenous to the South Sea Islands and was originally imported from there by European travelers. An interesting study in Germany in 1991 showed that anxiety in menopausal women significantly improved after one week of kava kava use.[25] Kava can be consumed as a beverage (as it is in the South Seas), but too much can cause over-sedation and mental impairment. This is rarely a problem with the standardized extracts in dosages of 100 mg three times a day. Kava should never be used in people with Parkinson's disease or those taking Valium or similar drugs. In rare instances, it has been associated with liver disease. Don't take kava and drive or do anything requiring quick reflexes until you determine how it will affect your system.

INSOMNIA AND FATIGUE

One of the most common complaints of menopause is a lack of restful sleep. Lack of restful sleep leads to fatigue the next day, which in turn leads to disrupted sleep the next night, and the cycle repeats. Eventually the sleeplessness is manifested as overall fatigue and moodiness.

Like many other problems, insomnia can have a multitude of causes. It is important, as with treating any of these problems, to work in concert with a trusted, competent medical professional to make sure there are no underlying problems. Many maladies, ranging from thyroid disorders, psychiatric conditions, and sleep apnea, can alter normal sleep. Be sure you are not just treating a symptom of an underlying non-hormonal disorder. Not all sleep problems in midlife are hormone related.

There is ample evidence that many of the sleep problems of menopause arise from the disruptive nature of hot flashes. You may experience hot flashes at night, which can wake you up several times and make going back to sleep that much more troublesome.

The obvious first approach to aiding sleep is to minimize the hot flashes. This alone can create blissful sleep for many with nightly heat surges. What if you have eliminated the night sweats (or never had them) and still have problems sleeping? What options are available other than potentially addictive sleeping pills?

God has provided many natural sleep aids that have proven effective. "People who work hard sleep well, whether they eat little or much. But the rich seldom get a good night's sleep" (Ecclesiastes 5:12). The writer of Ecclesiastes makes two important points about sleep. First, we know anecdotally and scientifically that exercise improves sleep. The Israelites knew it a long time ago. (For them it was not called exercise; it was called work.) If you are having a problem sleeping, get off your rear end and get active! It can't hurt, and it will help! That doesn't mean running a mile before bed. That would have just the opposite effect. But a healthy amount of activity during the day definitely promotes sleep. The second point made in the above verse is not that poor people sleep better than rich people, but that anxiety and worry are a leading cause of sleeplessness. A stress-filled day does not make for a relaxing night.

> The total direct costs in the United States for insomnia in 1995 were estimated to be $13.9 billion.[26]

Sleepy-Time Herbs

There are a few herbs that have been shown to help in promoting sleep. 5HTP has demonstrated in several double-blind studies to decrease the number of nighttime awakenings. A work published in 1988 reports that 5HTP not only aids in quantity of sleep but also in quality. The amount of REM, or rapid eye movement sleep, which is the most restful, is increased with 5HTP use.[27]

Valerian root (Valeriana officinalis) has been used for many years as a sedative and sleep aid. In 1982, a study was published that showed that valerian was able to improve the perceived quality of sleep in self-reported poor sleepers.[28] This was confirmed in a 1989 study where 89 percent reported improved sleep with the use of valerian.[29] A major plus for the use of valerian is the apparent lack of daytime drowsiness that can be associated with a traditional sleeping pill. The standard dose used in these studies is 1 to 3 grams about thirty minutes before bed. Be careful with valerian. If used properly and in appropriate doses it can be effective; however, it should not be used with any other prescription sleeping aids or benzodiazepines (Valium, Xanex, etc.).

The best-known complementary sleep aid is melatonin. Melatonin is a hormone secreted by the pineal gland, a small structure at the base of the brain. Unfortunately, the use of this hormone has been tainted by misinformation and media hype. There are a lot of shady operators in the natural medicine field, and none more so than in the promotion of melatonin. There is no question that melatonin has been shown to be a wonderful sleep aid, but only in people who have a low melatonin level.[30] Melatonin taken by people with normal levels (and that is the vast majority of us) will do little if anything for sleep, and may even backfire and disrupt sleep patterns. Women over the age of sixty have a higher likelihood of low melatonin, so they may experience some benefit from the substance. Before using this, see your doctor and be evaluated for its potential for effectiveness. Its most widely studied use is in balancing the sleep disturbances arising from jet lag.

> There are numerous causes of insomnia that can generally be broken down into three categories: (1) insomnia due to a sleep disorder, (2) insomnia due primarily to a physical medical disorder, and (3) insomnia due primarily to a psychiatric disorder.

You may be someone who suffers from leg cramps that keep you awake at night. One suggestion that has been successfully employed is bedtime magnesium tablets in a dose of 250–500 mg. There is also a new prescription medicine specifically for "restless legs syndrome."

There is good evidence that estrogen improves sleep, so if the benefits outweigh the risks, and all else has failed, consider HT to achieve restful sleep.

Treatment Summary for Insomnia and Fatigue

1. Reduce stress.
2. Eliminate hot flashes.
3. Exercise.

4. Take 5HTP (100 mg three times a day).

5. Use valerian root extract (1–3 grams one-half hour before bed).

6. Try melatonin if a deficiency exists.

7. Try bioidentical estradiol.

URINARY COMPLAINTS

"Every time I cough I wet my pants."

"I can't sing in the choir anymore because hitting the high notes means changing underwear."

"If I don't go right when I feel the urge, watch out. It's trouble."

"Even after I go I feel like I haven't fully emptied my bladder."

Studies state that 25-45% of women have suffered from incontinence at least once in the past year. The incidence of incontinence increases with age: 20–30% in young adults, 30–40% in the middle-aged, and as high as 50% in the elderly. One in three women who have had a baby experience some loss of bladder control.[31]

Have you ever experienced this embarrassment? Estimates say that over 13 million women in the United States suffer with some form of incontinence, the majority of which are perimenopausal. That translates into 33 percent of the population! What is staggering is that 50–70 percent of those affected don't tell their doctor about their problem and don't seek help. It is estimated that the health costs of incontinence amount to 20 billion dollars a year.

The message is twofold. One, you are not alone. Most people don't go to cocktail parties and sit around and say, "So, Marge, how is the dribbling?" It is a subject that is not talked about, but chances are someone close to you has a problem with urinary incontinence. Many women don't discuss it with their doctor because they are embarrassed or they think nothing can be done or they don't want any surgery or they feel it is a normal sign of aging. Poppycock to all those excuses!

Two, there is a lot that can be done for urinary incontinence both surgically and non-surgically. Understanding the physiology helps to understand your options. Urinary incontinence consists of four basic types: (1) anatomical droppage of the bladder—stress incontinence, (2) bladder spasms—detrusor instability, (3) a mixture of the two—the most common, and (4) overflow incontinence. Overflow incontinence is mainly limited to women with diabetes or selective neurological problems, and, since it is relatively rare, I won't spend much time discussing this type.

Stress incontinence is due to an anatomical drop in the bladder and is secondary to childbirth, aging, a loss of hormonal stimulation of the bladder and urethra, or a prior hysterectomy. It is treated in a variety of ways, but the majority involves a surgical correction of the bladder position (bladder tack). Contrast this with a bladder spasm (the second common type of incontinence, also known as an overactive bladder), which is treated mainly with behavioral modification and medication. Thus, identifying the type of incontinence is vital for you to choose the most effective treatment. Doing a bladder tack for bladder spasms will still leave you wet, and treating stress incontinence with medications will usually not solve that problem. The third category mentioned is a combination of both, and some estimates state that 60 to 75 percent of incontinent women have this mixture. In this instance, you must distinguish which type of incontinence is the predominant one. This will guide your therapy options. If you have a problem that is predominately bladder spasms, you can achieve adequate control from some medications and bladder retraining and never have to resort to surgery.

This topic is important because a substantial number of women in menopause suffer with incontinence. There is a pervasive myth that incontinence is just a part of aging. That is not the case. One of the first things you can do for this problem is have your hormonal status evaluated. The bladder and urethra are hormone-sensitive tissues, and urgency and incontinence may arise simply from a lack of estrogen stimulation. If that is the case, you can use some form of estrogen (creams, pills, etc.), and a few weeks to months later your bladder troubles markedly improve. It certainly is worth discussing with your doctor as part of your evaluation.

There are other methods to thwart stress urinary incontinence. One of the most useful is an exercise for the bladder. (I know you think I'm obsessed with exercise.) Many of you may already be familiar with Kegel exercises. When used consistently and persistently, they work! You may avoid surgery and maintain continence from doing these simple exercises.

The two biggest mistakes you may make are doing the exercises wrong or not being persistent.

The next time you are sitting on the commode, consciously stop your stream. The muscles that you tighten are the muscles you want to exercise. The idea is to contract these muscles and hold them for five seconds and then relax, and then repeat. Do this for five minutes three times a day, and you will see the benefits after a month. The wonderful thing about this exercise is no one knows you are doing anything. There are no special clothes to buy, no special machines needed, and you will never be annoyed by thirty-minute infomercials about them! Associate the need to do the Kegels with an already habitual event. For example, every time the phone rings, do your Kegels! (Use something different if you are a secretary or receptionist, or you may end up with a muscle-bound bladder!) It is not quick, but it will work. The alternatives are to live with it or to pay for a surgeon's new car by having an operation.

A related topic is cystitis, or bladder infections. This common female problem seems to be accentuated during menopause. This is largely due to a change in the normally acidic vaginal environment to a more basic one. This in turn leads to an alteration in the type and amount of bacteria in the vaginal canal. Because of the close anatomical relationship between the urethra and the vagina, it is easy for bacteria to migrate into the bladder where they are not welcome. This is the reason why intercourse is a predisposing reason for frequent bladder infections for some of you. In menopause, because of decreasing lubrication, you might experience a rise in the frequency of cystitis. There are some effective ways of not only treating these infections but also of preventing infections from ever invading.

First and foremost, you must drink adequate amounts of fluid. Drink a minimum of six to eight glasses of water a day. This is but a baseline; active people require much more. Water is ideal, but cranberry juice is helpful, especially for the bladder. Initially scientists speculated that it was the acid nature of the cranberry juice that exerted its protective effect; however, studies have shown that it is actually a substance in the juice that has antiseptic properties. A work done in 1991 published in the prestigious *New England Journal of Medicine* examined the beneficial effect of unsweetened cranberry juice and concluded it was effective at decreasing the frequency of urinary tract infections.[32]

Two other complementary approaches to preventing bladder infections involve the herbs uva-ursi (sounds like a constellation) and goldenseal. In 1993, Larsson and colleagues used a standardized 250 mg of uva-ursi in fifty-seven women with documented frequent urinary tract infections. The amazing results were that no women in the treatment group suffered a bout of cystitis for an entire year![33]

Goldenseal has long been known for its antibiotic-like effects. A study published in 1969 documented that the berberine in goldenseal was effective in treating uncomplicated urinary tract infections.[34] A word of caution: bladder infections by themselves are usually pretty harmless except for the discomfort they cause. However, if they go untreated or improperly treated, they could progress to a more serious infection. If you are using complementary methods of treating your cystitis, don't hesitate to contact your doctor if you are not seeing improvement in your symptoms within forty-eight hours. Complementary approaches are much more effective in preventing cystitis than treating it. Also, if you are in an immune-compromised situation such that infections may easily get out of control, don't hesitate to use the appropriate antibiotic to kill the infection at the outset.

Treatment Summary for Urinary Complaints

1. Discuss incontinence with your doctor, as it can't be helped if it is ignored.

2. Identify the type of incontinence (hard to do by yourself, see above).

3. Consider estradiol vaginal cream.

4. Eliminate caffeine. (Caffeine acts as a bladder irritant and can cause symptoms from frequency to urgency and even incontinence. I have seen many bladder symptoms disappear on a low- or no-caffeine diet.)

5. Do Kegel exercises.

6. Explore medication options.

7. Use surgical correction as a last resort for anatomical incontinence.

JOINT ACHES AND BODY ACHES

Laura was a bright, athletic woman in her late forties. She was menopausal, with the stopping of her periods one year prior. I enjoyed her visits because she, like me, was an avid distance runner. It would not be unusual for her to run thirty to forty miles a week. She had just finished her fourth marathon when she came for a routine checkup. Menopause had been little more than a blip on her screen, as she had experienced an occasional hot flash and that was it.

On this visit she said she was doing great except she was noticing some aches in her wrists and shoulders. They weren't severe, and she described them as a deep type of discomfort that didn't keep her from doing things (obviously), but was nagging. I initially wrote it off as being a residual effect from her recent marathon. I told her to get plenty of rest and decrease her mileage over the next month. If it didn't get better, come and see me then. A month passed, and I had forgotten our discussion when I saw her running on the riverbank one Saturday morning. We ran together for a while, and she said she had fully recovered from the race and was only doing two- to three-mile runs, but the discomfort she had described earlier was still there. From her description I suspected an orthopedic problem, so I set up a referral with a colleague the next week.

I spoke to her a few weeks later and found out that he had put her through a whole battery of tests and could find nothing to explain her pain. She was taking Motrin and it helped, but she was concerned that she was treating a symptom and not a cause.

It just so happened that I spent the next weekend in Atlanta at a conference on complementary approaches to common health problems, and one of the presenters had talked about the "body ache, bone pain" syndrome of menopause. He stated that many women will experience this nonspecific ache in any bone or joint in the body, and this was thought to be secondary to the decreased lubrication and secretions of the joint space. This sounded amazingly like Laura's situation, so when I got back, I called her and discussed what I had learned. The first thing she did was increase her dietary phytoestrogens. Then she added some estradiol cream. Within two weeks she was noticing some improvement, but she didn't feel she was there yet.

I then suggested glucosamine sulfate. Glucosamine is a naturally occurring substance that plays an important role in the biochemistry of cartilage; in particular, it serves as the basic building block of glycosaminoglycans, which are essential components of cartilage. Glucosamine sulfate has been studied extensively for treating osteoarthritis and has been shown to have an anti-inflammatory effect. A large multicentered trial in France compared the efficacy of glucosamine with that of a prescription nonsteroidal anti-inflammatory medicine, Piroxicam. They found that glucosamine was significantly more effective than the Piroxicam and placebo in relief of joint pain.[35] The presenter at the conference had taken this data and used the glucosamine in his menopausal patients with these diffuse, nebulous joint discomforts. His results were impressive, so I felt it was worth a try with Laura.

Within a month she was pain free and running better than ever! Since then, I have used this regimen and found it to be very helpful in almost everyone with these particular "achy" complaints. The most researched dose is 500 mg three times a day. Studies have also documented the safety and lack of significant side effects. The literature is full of reports of glucosamine sulfate and its potent analgesic effects, especially on bone and joint pain. I must stress that it is critical to rule out various other causes of joint and bone pain before assuming it is hormone related. Get a proper physical and, if all else appears normal, consider this wonderful solution.

Treatment Summary for Joint Aches and Body Aches

1. Rule out other medical conditions.

2. Take glucosamine sulfate for joint and bone pain (500 mg three times a day).

3. Exercise.

4. Increase dietary phytoestrogens.

5. Try therapeutic massage.

BOUNCING, BINGEING, BONES, AND BELIEVING

ॐ

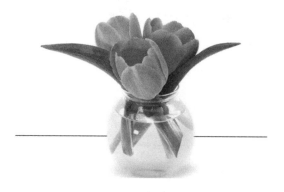

EXERCISE: SWEATING WITH THE OLDIES

Exercise is not an option! Immutable Rule #3: If you don't use it, you're going to lose it!

The third "A" in the prescription for success in menopause is *action*. If your goal is to live a healthy, long, happy life, exercise is not a maybe! It must be a part of your daily routine. There are multitudes of benefits, and the intensity and duration needed to achieve these benefits can be adapted to almost any situation.

What else can help you feel better, look better, act better, lower cholesterol, reduce fat, strengthen your heart, decrease osteoporosis, improve PMS, treat depression, boost the immune system, increase libido, improve sleep, build self-esteem—and is cheap? There is nothing else on the planet that can accomplish all this, and with no side effects to boot! God has designed the perfect fountain of youth, and it is available to all, regardless of age or current health. But you have to drink from it for thirty to forty minutes daily for it to work!

God designed us to move. Every muscle, bone, and tendon is geared for motion. The rewards of inactivity include obesity, breathlessness, multiple medications, and depression. Proverbs 19:24 says, "Lazy people take food in their hand but don't even lift it to their mouth." Not a good exercise plan or weight loss diet.

The choice is yours!

EXERCISE IS BIBLICAL

The Bible, especially the New Testament, is filled with analogies to athletics and physical activities. Paul's letters in particular employ physical activity imagery to drive home important spiritual points. I think it is intentional that these references appear frequently, and they underscore the importance of exercise in a balanced lifestyle. Paul writes in 1 Corinthians,

> Don't you realize that in a race everyone runs, but only one person gets the prize? So run to win! All athletes are disciplined in their training. They do it to win a prize that will fade away, but we do it for an eternal prize. So I run with purpose in every step. I am not just shadowboxing. I discipline my body like an athlete, training it to do what it should. Otherwise, I fear that after preaching to others I myself might be disqualified. (9:24–27)

Philippians 3:14 says, "I press on to reach the end of the race and receive the heavenly prize for which God, through Christ Jesus, is calling us." In 2 Timothy 4:7-8, Paul writes, "I have fought the good fight, I have finished the race, and I have remained faithful. And now the prize awaits me—the crown of righteousness, which the Lord, the righteous Judge, will give me on the day of his return. And the prize is not just for me but for all who eagerly look forward to his appearing." And Hebrews 12:1 says, "Therefore, since we are surrounded by such a huge crowd of witnesses to the life of faith, let us strip off every weight that slows us down, especially the sin that so easily trips us up. And let us run with endurance the race God has set before us."

MARATHON

This is an area where I practice what I preach. To date I have run eleven marathons, and I hope to do many more. Isaiah 40:28–31 inspired me and helped me survive my first marathon.

Have you never heard? Have you never understood? The Lord is the everlasting God, the Creator of all the earth. He never grows weak or weary. No one can measure the depths of his understanding. He gives power to the weak and strength to the powerless. Even youths will become weak and tired, and young men will fall in exhaustion. But those who trust in the Lord will find new strength. They will soar high on wings like eagles. They will run and not grow weary. They will walk and not faint.

This was my prayer as I rounded the turn and entered the final miles of the twenty-six-mile race on the hills of San Francisco. I am convinced that without these verses to motivate me, I may not have completed that run. Whether it is running a race, making a decision, surviving an emotional heartbreak, or conquering a mental challenge, God is there to provide motivation and guidance. I repeated this verse hundreds of times in my training runs and meditated on it in the actual race.

Paul puts exercise in perspective in his letter to Timothy: "Physical training is good, but training for godliness is much better, promising benefits in this life and in the life to come" (1 Timothy 4:8). There is no question that physical exercise is beneficial, yet the focus is balance. You can let exercise become an obsession, quickly turning it into an idol. Balance mind, body, and spirit.

Excuses not to exercise are as abundant as politicians on the take. "But, Doc, I don't have time to exercise!" Translated, this really means, "I don't want to make time to exercise." Every time a patient uses that excuse, I challenge her. Her office visit will be free if I can't find at least three ten minute-segments in her daily schedule in which she can undertake some form of useful exercise. (Studies indicate that a short time frame can be beneficial to start with.) And I tell folks I will not ask them to do anything that I won't or haven't done myself. I haven't given away a single office visit yet. (My office manager cringes every time I do this.)

I also frequently hear, "But, Doc, I'm sixty years old and have never exercised; what good will it do me now?"

The answer is simple—a great deal. If your doctor says you can (and I would question him/her if they said otherwise), there is much to be gained from an exercise regimen tailored to your needs and abilities. If your only exercise is jumping to conclusions, don't stagger out the door tomorrow and run a mile. If you do that, make sure your companion knows CPR! Get proper advice from your doctor about what you can do (focus on that instead of what you can't do), and start slow. In this instance, being a turtle is much more advantageous than being a rabbit. But the message is, "Just do it." Start today!

You are never too old to exercise. A study published a few years back looked at ninety-year-old men and their ability to benefit from weight-bearing exercise. These were folks in various levels of health, and they were guided through individualized routines for six weeks. Universally the men showed improvement in strength and muscle mass. They all said they felt and slept better. One fellow said it had revived his sex life! Excuses don't work, and age is not a limiting factor. The only limiting factor is the muscle between your ears!

> Medical experts warn that compulsive exercising can be just as bad for a person as no exercise at all. The human body needs 24 hours without exercise about once a week in order to cleanse itself of lactic acid and other waste products of strenuous activity.

Maya Angelou said, "Lift up your hearts. Each new hour holds new chances for new beginnings." If it is no more than walking up and down stairs, do something. The shelves are full of good manuals on everything from active stretching to power walking. Get a good checkup, pick something you like doing, and for your sake, do it!

An exercise regimen must be individualized. Just because Uncle Harry ran his first marathon at sixty-five doesn't mean you have to match him step for step. It also doesn't mean you can't! Too many times people begin by asking, "What are the things I shouldn't be doing?" The real question is, what *can* I do?

WHY EXERCISE?

You must educate yourself about your body. The more you know, the better decisions you make. Learning basic physiology of exercise and metabolism is important because it forms the foundation for understanding and motivating you to "move to the groove"!

What happens when you exercise? Why is all this stuff helpful? How can I amaze and bedazzle my friends at parties with my knowledge of metabolism? The answers are simple. So simple, we tend to forget them right after high school biology class. What follows is a quick primer in menopausally relevant physiology. I can feel the excitement building!

> "There are more than 630 muscles in your body. On average, your body weight is 40% muscle.... The muscles surrounding your eye are the busiest muscles in your body. Research indicates that you probably blink them more than 100,000 times a day."[1]

FAT

Fat, blubber, jelly belly, love handles, spare tire, thunder thighs—all identify the same condition, being over fat. We can all agree that fat is a problem for most of us. Well, fat is actually your friend! The only problem is that most of us get too much of a good thing. You have heard of overstaying your welcome. When it comes to fat, many of us have allowed the guests to move in permanently!

Fat was deliberately put in our bodies by God not as punishment but as a phenomenal energy source. When we spend time exercising, we begin to tell the fat cells to give up some of that important fuel. After about twenty or thirty minutes of exercise, the muscles scream for more energy, and our intuitively wise body responds by dipping into its fat reserves for a highly concentrated and efficient source of fuel. We "release the grease," as Covert Bailey says in his book *Smart Exercise*.[2]

To put it simply, if we exert ourselves in short bursts (like chasing the two-year-old around the house, or cleaning the bathroom), we tend to selectively burn sugar (glucose). This sugar is readily available and easily metabolized, so it is the first choice when the activity is relatively short-lived. However, if the energy expenditure extends over a longer period of time, the body calls on its reserves, primarily fat, and begins to burn this for fuel. When fat is metabolized, your thighs get smaller and your belly becomes flatter!

The secret to efficient fat burning is making the exercise *aerobic* and *sustained.* Aerobic means with oxygen, and this element is absolutely essential in the metabolism of fat.

> Only muscles burn fat, and active muscles are the most efficient way to change your metabolism.

Your level of fitness is literally how well your muscles burn oxygen. A simple way of determining whether your exercise is aerobic is to measure your pulse while exercising, and if it is elevated above 110, you are doing something right. However, and this is just as important, you should always be able to carry on a conversation while exercising. If you are too out of breath to do this, you have to slow down and build up to that level more slowly. Many people use fancy heart-rate monitors to check their exercise intensity. Save your dollars and instead simply take your pulse for six seconds and multiply by ten, and there you have your beats per minute!

The second component to fat-burning aerobic exercise is sustained activity. Studies show that to attain maximal fat burning, you must exercise aerobically for a minimum of twenty minutes. Fat burning is not the only goal of exercise. Exercise changes your body chemistry to make it healthier the other twenty-three hours of the day you are not exercising. There are many things you can do that will build strength, protect bones, and contribute to overall health other than aerobic exercise. Weight lifting is rarely an aerobic exercise, but it can be very beneficial to women in menopause, especially when dealing with osteoporosis prevention. Pilates and stretching are great exercises, yet they are rarely aerobic.

To prevent stagnation and achieve overall physical health, consider alternating activities. This common practice, called cross-training, is the quickest, most enjoyable way of achieving and maintaining fitness. For example, on Monday go for a brisk forty-five-minute walk. Tuesday spend a half-hour lifting weights. Wednesday play golf (no carts and walk fast). Thursday do Pilates or stretching. Friday take another good walk. Saturday can be a second weight session, and Sunday you rest and thank God for letting you do all that stuff during the week!

Keys to efficient exercise

ᔄ Wind sprints: Increase the velocity of your pace for 30 seconds several times during your walk.

ᔄ Aerobic exercise burns fat. Do something where you don't gasp for breath.

ᔄ Lift weights to build muscle…to burn fat.

ᔄ Cross-train. Don't do the same thing every day. Alter your routines.

THE SECRET TO WEIGHT LOSS

Some eternal truths are painful to acknowledge. One of those is that when you take in more calories than you burn up, you gain weight. When you burn up more than you take in, you lose weight. This is a basic rule of nature, like "What goes up must come down." It is unalterable regardless of the imagery, positive thinking, or medications employed. Positive thinking may help your attitude, but it won't change your fitness level.

Billions of dollars are spent each year instructing people on the best ways of losing weight. When you break down every single workable method to its most basic components, it is either a way of decreasing intake (diet) or increasing output (exercise). All the prescription and natural medications available are designed to either help you eat less or attempt to fool your body into burning up more. No matter how fancy the name or how sophisticated the machine, all weight control plans fall into one of these two categories.

A common misperception is that there is a relationship between being thin and being healthy. That is not the case. I know many sick, skinny people and several chubby, healthy folks. Granted you have a greater likelihood of medical problems if you are overweight; however, the gauge of your health does not solely depend on your bathroom scale. Health is much more than simply the absence of disease. Remember, it is a joyful balance; your body contour doesn't necessarily paint an accurate picture of your state of health. For example, you are much better off being twenty pounds overweight and leading an active lifestyle than at ideal body weight and smoking a pack of cigarettes a day. It is easy to equate weight with health—it's so visual! But dress size is only part of the equation. Let me say emphatically here, sustainable weight loss and fitness can only be achieved with exercise as a part of the total program.

OVERWEIGHT VERSUS OVER FAT

To tie the idea of weight, health, and fat together, consider the two terms *overweight* and *over fat*. "What's the difference?" you ask.

The difference is that you can be over fat and be normal weight! For you non-exercisers this is a scary concept. Take Eloise, a forty-two-year-old woman who is 5'8" and weighs 128 pounds. She has worn the same dress size since college. She is proud that she can still wear her cheerleading outfit from high school (although I don't know why she'd want to). The problem with Eloise is not her weight but her body fat. When she was eighteen she was extremely active and exercised excessively. She weighed about 128 then, but if you compared the amount of muscle that made up her weight, you would have found that about 78 percent of her weight was lean body mass (muscle and bone). This gave her about 22 percent body fat. This is considered very healthy for women. As she aged, Eloise became less active and her muscle mass declined. If you look at unused muscles under the microscope, you can actually see little fat cells that become deposited in the muscle. So after several years of decreased activity, Eloise is still 128 pounds, but her body fat has climbed to 42 percent. This leads to a corresponding drop in her lean body mass (muscle).

STEALTH OBESITY

Why is this important? You can become over fat and not realize the risk to your health. It is stealth obesity. It is there, but it is not detected before the damage is done. Many will become over fat before they become overweight.

Being over fat is a risk factor for heart disease, stroke, diabetes, and obesity. If you can avoid being over fat, then you can avoid many of the health problems that are associated with external obesity. If you are overweight, it is something you can see (all too well). It is only natural to identify outwardly visible obesity as the bad guy. If you really want to make a difference, you need to focus on how to become unfat! The goal is to be healthy, not just thin.

How do you get unfat, or ideally, prevent yourself from ever getting fat in the first place? You guessed it! Exercise. (See how all this ties together?) Exercise is not only for losing weight. The goal of exercise is to get your body moving to provide an internal environment that is optimal for your good health.

The external appearance is a nice by-product, but your focus should be on the inside. It is not necessarily the outward appearance that is the trophy; it is the internal change that holds the promise for your good health and longevity. At the most basic level, exercise improves both physical and mental health, especially in midlife.

American Obesity Epidemic

- Fifty-eight million adults are overweight; 40 million obese; 3 million morbidly obese.

- Six out of 10 persons over 25 are overweight.

- Seventy-eight percent of Americans are not meeting basic activity level recommendations.

- There has been a 76% increase in Type 2 diabetes in adults 30 to 40 years old since 1990.[3]

PERCENT BODY FAT

No doubt you all have seen the charts extolling the virtue of obtaining your "ideal body weight." These charts have done for you about as much disservice as the media's glamorization of the "ideal woman." The charts are inaccurate reminders of an inappropriate measurement of health. Body weight is not the best parameter to follow if you are truly interested in health. Weight is easy to measure, and there is a correlation between risk factors and weight. So in that respect, the charts are peripherally useful. But given a choice, knowing your percent body fat is a much more valuable tool in assessing your health. Unfortunately it is much more difficult to get accurate measurements of body fat percentage than weight.

The best way to check your body fat is to be weighed in a water tank while submerged. The underwater immersion test is the most accurate measure, and it is the method used most often by universities and physiology labs when doing research. Not many of us can drive down the street to our friendly immersion tank and get our body fat calculated once a month, so several simpler methods of estimating body fat percentage have been developed.

Covert Bailey, in *Smart Exercise*, talks about a simple method you can use at your next swimming party. It's based on the fact that fat floats and muscle sinks. Have all your guests float on their backs in the pool. Have them take a deep breath and, when prompted, blow it all out. His informal research has shown that above 25 percent body fat, people float easily. At 22 to 23 percent fat, one can float while breathing shallowly. At 15 percent body fat, one will usually sink slowly even with the lungs full of air. And at 13 percent body fat, one will sink readily with a chest full of air, even in salt water![4] This is a fun way to get a basic idea of body fat.

A more accurate determination is using a skin caliper. It is a small, simple device that a trained person can use to grasp a skin fold, say in your upper arm, and measure the thickness. A formula can then be used to calculate the correct percent of body fat. If done properly, this can be an amazingly accurate measure of your body fat percentage. Many doctors offer these measurements in their offices, and most health clubs and gyms have someone on staff who can perform this quick and easy test. Some machines that check bone density can also assess total body fat. Next time you go in for a bone densiometry, ask about getting your body fat assessed. There are now some relatively inexpensive scales for home use that measure percent body fat by using electric measurements. They are accurate and give you a better sense of your fitness than relying solely on weight. The ideal body fat percentage for guys is around 15 percent and for midlife women around 25 percent. The average (measured from thousands of people) is 25 percent for men and 33 percent for women.

If you want a practical, livable, simple guide to fat control for the whole family, check out my book *Fat-Proof Your Family* (shameless plug).

Walking—The Perfect Exercise?

∞ Walking is free and requires no special equipment or training.

∞ Almost everyone is capable of walking.

∞ You can walk almost anywhere.

∞ Walking is safe and low-impact, with a low risk of injuries and accidents.

∞ Walking for health can be combined easily with walking for other reasons.

∞ You can enjoy a variety of surroundings as you walk in different places and different seasons.

∞ You don't need to concentrate on the walking itself, leaving you free to enjoy your surroundings, chat to companions, or just relax.[5]

WHERE DO I START?

Okay, so you are convinced that exercise is a good thing. "Well, Exercise Boy," you ask, "where do I start?" For those of you whose idea of exercise is clicking the TV remote control, the place to start is with your doctor. Before you begin any new activity, it is a grand idea to get a good checkup. Ask your doctor for guidelines. Ask how to start and what exercises would be good for you. If your doctor says you can't do at least some form of exercise, I would get a second opinion.

Almost everyone can begin a walking program. There are some obvious exceptions, but there are even options for those who can't walk. Numerous research studies indicate that walking is one of the best forms of exercise. Start slowly, and gradually build up both your time spent walking and your speed. Remember, the importance of aerobic exercise is to help eliminate fat. To be aerobic, exercise must be swift enough to elevate your heart rate but not so fast that you can't continue to have a conversation while walking. You don't want to be pushing so hard as to be gasping for breath. This level of exertion will vary based on your level of fitness and previous experience with walking. My wife walks as her primary fitness tool, but it is not a Sunday stroll through the park. She can cover a mile walking faster than I can running! Now, that may say more about the speed at which I run, but it illustrates that walking can be an aerobic experience!

The secret to any exercise program is to start slowly and build. Each week increase either your intensity or time spent in exercise. When you have peaked in those areas, look for more challenging terrain. A hill here and there can really spice up an otherwise tedious walk. Bring along a friend. If you are like me and like exercise to be personal time, use it wisely for prayer or just clearing your head. You will be amazed at how many problems are unintentionally solved and how spiritual this time can be.

There are a few guidelines that will make your exercise routine more efficient and effective. First, throw away the pedometer and get a watch. Whether you are walking, running, doing aerobics, swimming, or rock climbing, it is the time involved and not the distance that matters. In other words, walk forty-five minutes instead of four miles. Studies show that it is the time, not the mileage, that burns fat and improves cardiovascular systems. In the real world, pace and effort can vary, so time spent in the activity is the most important factor in determining cardiovascular benefit.

If you want to accelerate the benefit, increase the time spent in the activity. Increasing intensity or speed will burn fat quicker, but you still have to put in the time to get the maximum benefit. There is some recent research that reports the cardiovascular benefit of exercise can be obtained by doing brief periods (ten minutes) of vigorous activity two to three times a day instead of all at once. This will certainly help the heart muscle, but it is not the most efficient way to burn fat. How do you know if you are walking at a rate that will benefit your cardiovascular health and burn fat? Take your pulse! Your heartbeat should be elevated, and stay that way, in a range of 65 percent to 80 percent of its calculated maximum. (See Table 9.)

TABLE 9: CALCULATION OF MAXIMUM HEART RATE

220 minus your age = maximum heart rate (applies if you don't have heart disease and are not on medications that affect heart rate)

65 to 80% of maximum heart rate = recommended training range

Example: 50-year-old woman with no heart disease, maximum heart rate would be 220-50 = 170. Recommended training heart rate would be 111–136.

Your breathing should be deep, but you shouldn't be gasping for air; again, you should be able to carry on a conversation while exercising. Record your results. Keep a log of your activity and times. This will help you evaluate your progress and motivate you to continue.

Here are a few common forms of exercise that, when done at the proper level of intensity, are aerobic: walking, running, bicycling, stationary biking, rowing, cross-country skiing, swimming, stair climbing, hiking, treadmill walking, roller-skating, ice-skating, in-line skating, class aerobics, bench aerobics, water aerobics, yelling at teenagers (just kidding).

What may be surprising to you is the list of activities that are not usually aerobic. But it doesn't mean these activities are not useful, since any movement is better than no movement.

The following activities usually don't provide the *continual* heart rate elevation necessary to achieve aerobic benefit: tennis, golf, handball, racquetball, line dancing, softball, weight lifting, and sex (the intensity may be there, but usually not the duration). These provide excellent cross-training or off-day activities, but don't expect nine holes of golf three times a week to keep you fit and trim. Mix and match activities from both groups to avoid boredom and to keep your muscles fooled. An ideal health program encourages you to do something aerobic three days a week for a minimum of thirty minutes, and then a non-aerobic activity on the alternate days.

REST

Rest is an essential component of any exercise program. It is actually during the rest times that muscle is built and repaired. A fit person's body is burning more calories than that of a non-fit person, even at rest!

As you build your lean body mass (muscle), you increase the number of calories required to maintain that muscle. So even when you are sleeping, your fit body is burning more fuel to maintain and repair the often-used muscles.

Most of us won't have to worry about overtraining, but keep in mind that rest is critical to continuing injury-free exercise. God knew the importance of rest. "On the seventh day God had finished his work of creation, so he rested from all his work" (Genesis 2:2).

THUNDER THIGHS

Not long ago Millie came to me after a conference presentation and said, "All this about exercise is good and nice, and I even buy in to the idea of it being good for me. But I want to know how to get rid of my thunder thighs and my cellulite."

First, I told her not to waste money on rubs or creams—all those do is reduce the water content of the tissues, and that will bounce right back. Second, I explained the reasons behind that ugly fat. In a woman, this type of fat lies right under the skin and is called subcutaneous fat. It is deposited first on the inside of the thigh, then on the outside of the thigh. Then the fat is placed on the hips, the torso, and then the upper body, mainly the area under the arms. This is a fact of female physiology, and it probably is a result of God's design to maximize the childbearing and nourishing ability of the female. How much goes to each area, and how quickly it gets there, are genetically determined. (Thanks, Mom!) For the majority of women, these fat deposits are removed in the reverse order when fat is lost. In other words, as you begin fat-burning exercise, the first deposits to come off are the upper body and arms, followed by the torso and so on. The last bastion of fat is those thighs.

Spot-reducing is a fantasy. It just doesn't happen. If you see someone who has recently started an exercise program and one week later their hips and thighs are noticeably smaller, I would check their medical bills, because it is likely they have paid a visit to their neighborhood plastic surgeon. To get rid of the thunder thighs and cellulite, you must do aerobic exercise consistently and for whatever time it takes. For some it may be weeks; for others, months. There is no quick fix. Accept it, and get off your fanny and do something good for yourself.

Dr. George Sheehan, physician, author, and runner, said, "The choice is for fitness or fatness, to exercise or not to exercise. The ultimate cure for obesity is exercise."[6]

EXERCISE: A TOOL FOR HEALING

The main goals for exercise and fitness are to live better and prevent physical and emotional illness. Have you ever thought of exercise as a tool for healing? What about using exercise like you would a drug or a bandage? We are familiar with the use of exercise in the rehabilitation of heart attack patients. Everyone marvels at the physical therapy and devotion of the injured athlete striving to regain the competitive edge. What about the everyday aches and pains and common ills that strike us? Can exercise be a healing influence? Sure it can. Let's look at how.

Aging

Exercise is the fountain of youth. Dr. William Simpson, researcher on aging and professor of Family Medicine at the Medical University of South Carolina, states, "If we stay active many of the things that supposedly decline with age really don't decline."[7]

One of the most prevalent myths of aging is that older people don't need or benefit from exercise. Numerous studies point to just the opposite conclusion. Light to moderate exercise, even in a ninety-year-old, can delay aging. More important, it will improve the quality of life. A National Institute of Aging survey showed that only 27 percent of people over sixty-five exercise regularly.[8] With those over sixty-five being the fastest-growing segment of the population today, it is critically important that these folks (and we will all be these folks sooner or later) be taught the benefits of exercise and be motivated to participate.

Will regular exercise help you live longer at a better quality of life? Yes, and once again science supports this. In a study of over sixteen thousand Harvard graduates followed over sixteen years, those who exercised moderately on a daily basis had a 33 percent lower death rate than their couch potato counterparts. A newsletter from the Baylor College of Medicine said, "The most exhausting part of exercising is the mental argument that takes place when you try to talk yourself into getting up off the couch and just doing it!"[9]

Arthritis

Years ago doctors prescribed excessive rest for people struggling with osteoarthritis. The only problem with this regimen was that people consistently got worse rather than better. The approach to arthritis today is dramatically different. Studies over the past ten years have shown that simple exercise, such as walking and swimming, can be extremely therapeutic. Exercise can increase strength and flexibility and, for some, allow them to cut back on their medications. Age and degree of arthritis doesn't appear to be a limiting factor. Dr. Donald Kay, who treats many arthritis patients, said, "Even people in their mid-eighties have improved with exercise."[10]

The continued functioning of the joints, especially diseased joints, depends on their movement. Moving the joints increases the production of synovial fluid, the lubricant so essential in smooth joint operation. It also increases blood flow, which in turn reduces inflammation. Swimming has been identified as one of the best exercises if you are bothered by arthritis because of its low impact on the joints and its great range of motion capabilities. The growth of water aerobics programs around the country is testament to their effectiveness.

This is an area where you must develop an exercise program in concert with your doctor. There are rare types of bone and joint problems where exercise may not be as valuable, and you must have some parameters as far as intensity and type of exercise undertaken. See your doctor, jump in the pool, and put the Motrin on the shelf!

Constipation

Most people will experience this annoying problem occasionally, while some are afflicted on a regular or chronic basis. The secret to avoiding constipation is fiber, fluid, and fartlek. We will cover fiber and fluid in the chapter on diet. If you are not sure you are getting enough fiber or fluids, you probably aren't. *Fartlek* is a Swedish word familiar to most runners that means "speed play." Here I use it to represent any exercise.

Studies have actually looked at the transit time of food in the bowels and have discovered that people who exercise have a quicker rate of food passage. Many scientists believe that the faster transit time in exercisers is due to an increased secretion of hormones that stimulate bowel action. Sit-ups, or any activity that increases the strength of the abdominal muscles, can enhance the passage of food in the intestines and can make its expulsion easier. An eighty-year-old lady gave me some advice several years back and I have never forgotten it. She said, "Honey, at my age, if my bowels are happy, I'm happy!"

Varicose Veins

I hate to disappoint you, but exercise will not get rid of the bothersome roadmap veins. What it can do is help prevent them from getting any worse, and, in some women, keep them from coming up at all. Varicosities are nothing more than dilated blood vessels. They arise secondary to the weakening of the vessel wall or due to stasis of the blood. Exercise gets the blood pumping and forces the vessels to be more efficient at emptying. Some people may develop worse veins if they exercise and don't wear support hose, so check with your doctor.

"About 50 to 55% of American women and 40 to 45% of American men suffer from some form of vein problem. Varicose veins affect 1 out of 2 people age 50 and older."[11]

Memory

Have you ever walked into a room and couldn't remember why you were there? Have you forgotten someone's name that you had known for twenty years? Research has shown that even these common memory lapses can be helped by regular exercise. A study done at Ohio State University took seventy-two people (average age of sixty-three) and had them ride stationary bikes three times a week for nine months. The researchers found that exercise improved attention span, concentration, and short-term memory.[12]

Robert Dustman, PhD, published a study from the VA hospital in Salt Lake City that showed a group of people between the ages of fifty-five and seventy improved their memory and other cognitive measures by participating in a brisk walking program. He compared these patients with non-exercisers and a group that just used weights and did stretching. The walkers showed significant improvement over both groups.[13] Evidence shows that active people have a keener sense of visual recall. Some scientists have speculated that regular exercise increases the blood flow to the brain, and this may be responsible for the improved cognitive functioning.

Have you gotten the message yet? I think now you may better understand my admonition at the beginning of this chapter that exercise is not an option! There are unlimited types of activities that can be used for exercise—from sitting in a chair lifting cans of soup to joining a local health club and becoming a gym rat. And there is always time. If you don't make time to exercise, then you will have to make time to be sick.

Action Challenge

1. Get a good physical exam.

2. Get started today.

3. Do something aerobic at least three times a week.

4. Make it fun and something you enjoy.

5. Exercise with a partner or group for accountability.

6. Be consistent and persistent.

7. Reap the benefits!

DIET AND NUTRITION: EAT SMART—LIVE LONG

How many times have you heard the old adage, "You are what you eat"? If you are like me, probably too many times. It often emanates from the mouth of a twig-sized Spandex workout queen who never had a weight problem in her life. Your first inclination is to waddle up to her and stuff tofu in her ear. But being the Christian woman that you are, you fight this temptation and smile and say, "Well, I guess that makes me a Butterball turkey!"

The unfortunate thing about so many old adages is that many are true. And this is one of them. The fuel that we put into our bodies is the building block for every molecule, organ, and thought we have. The good news is that healthy dietary habits can have a positive impact on your midlife body and soul.

SAD (STANDARD AMERICAN DIET)

We are a nation of poor eaters. Some studies estimate that over 60 percent of the adult population can be categorized as overweight.

Fifteen to 40 percent of *children* are overweight.[1] The nutritional habits that are formed in the early years influence us throughout our lives. Although you are past childhood, many of you have a child or teenager who respects your opinion (I realize including teenagers here is stretching reality), and you can have a major impact on their nutritional habits. Your two most powerful teaching tools are the grocery cart and your example. You or your spouse buys the food that comes into the house. Granted, many kids eat at school and may have only one meal at home, but what constitutes that meal and how it is prepared is your choice. This can't be a "Do as I say and not as I do" lesson. You must model good eating habits for those habits to have an impact on those around you. Studies indicate that the mother in a household is the single most influential person regarding the overall health of the family.

Consider the health problems related to poor dietary practices. Heart disease, diabetes, stroke, cancer, and joint and bone problems are just a few of the maladies that are largely environmental—their occurrence is markedly influenced by the choices you make. Adhering to a few simple dietary guidelines can dramatically reduce the incidence of all these problems.

NORMAL IS NOT HEALTHY

The standard American diet (SAD) that has been preached for years is fraught with myths, misperceptions, and downright lies. When it comes to food, you need to think abnormally! Normal is not necessarily healthy. If you strive to achieve the average daily allowances of calories and nutrients, the average intake of fats, carbohydrates, and proteins, and the average cholesterol, then you will probably have the average heart attack, the average stroke, or the average spare tire! Think abnormally; strive for what is truly healthy, not what is average. Don't fall into the trap of complacency by limiting yourself to "good enough" when it comes to your diet.

Nutrition Questionnaire[2]

Read the statements below. Circle the number in the "yes" column for those that apply to you.

	YES
I have an illness or condition that made me change the kind and/or amount of food I eat.	2
I eat fewer than two meals per day.	3
I eat few fruits or vegetables or milk products.	2
I have three or more drinks of beer, liquor, or wine almost every day.	2
I have tooth or mouth problems that make it hard for me to eat.	2
I don't always have enough money to buy the food I need.	4
I eat alone most of the time.	1
I take three or more different prescribed or over-the-counter drugs a day.	1
Without wanting to, I have lost or gained ten pounds in the last six months.	2
I am not always physically able to shop, cook, and/or feed myself.	2
TOTAL	

Total the numbers you have circled. If your nutritional score is

0-2	Good! Recheck your nutritional score in six months.
3-5	You are at moderate nutritional risk. See what can be done to improve your eating habits and lifestyle.
6 or more	You are at high nutritional risk. Bring this checklist the next time you see your doctor. Ask for help to improve your nutritional health.

WHAT THE BIBLE SAYS

"Don't you realize that your body is the temple of the Holy Spirit, who lives in you and was given to you by God? You do not belong to yourself, for God bought you with a high price. So you must honor God with your body" (1 Corinthians 6:19–20).

Paul, in his letter to the Corinthians, says that what you do with your body is important. You are not free to treat your body any way you please. That is a gross misinterpretation of free will. Your physical body, along with your spirit, belongs to God. *The Life Application Bible* commentary points out, "When we become Christians, the Holy Spirit comes to live in us. Therefore, we no longer own our bodies. That God bought us 'with a high price' refers to slaves purchased at an auction. Christ's death freed us from sin but also obligates us to His service. If you live in a building owned by someone else, you try not to violate the building's rules. Because your body belongs to God, you must not violate His standards for living. So many of the problems that we encounter in health and illness are due to not obeying the instructions of God."[3]

Granted there are many symptoms of menopause and many illnesses of advanced age that are totally unrelated to diet and lifestyle; however, a survey of the leading causes of death in this country—heart disease, stroke, and cancer—quickly shows that we are still doing something wrong.

Our longevity has dramatically improved over time, but much of that increase is due to the successful treatment of infectious diseases and improvement in public health and hygiene. We continue to have a major problem with lifestyle diseases such as heart disease, stroke, and some cancers. Christians are called to respect the temple (body), and it is obvious that the consequences of not doing so are great.

Now the Good News

I don't want to paint a doom and gloom picture, because there is a great deal of good news on healthy living and healthy eating. Thankfully, it doesn't involve eating only kelp casseroles and cardboard cereal! God didn't put you here without specific instructions on how to fuel this "temple of the Holy Spirit." That would be like giving you a new car but not telling you what it takes to make it go. Putting syrup in the gas tank will clog up the engine. That is essentially what a lot of people do! They put all this garbage into their system and expect it to run like a Swiss watch. Wouldn't it make more sense to simply read the instructions? I admit that I am one of those people who rarely reads instructions, and I have a gadget graveyard to prove it. This is not smart or efficient. New computer software comes with a "Read Me" file. The "Read Me" file for your internal computer is the Bible! So what does the Bible say about healthy eating?

A Holy Healthy Smorgasbord

God created specific substances for food. Look at Genesis chapter 1, verses 29–30: "Then God said, 'Look! I have given you every seed-bearing plant throughout the earth and all the fruit trees for your food. And I have given every green plant as food for all the wild animals, the birds in the sky, and the small animals that scurry along the ground—everything that has life.'"

This is not too tough to figure out. God says that a predominately vegetarian diet is healthy. These are the perfect foods! Anyone who is familiar with current nutritional research can tell you a diet based on fruits, vegetables, and plants is by far the most beneficial to one's health. Balance is the key. God designed and provided an enormous variety of foods for a reason. I believe it is to give an almost limitless supply of the various nutrients we need to optimally function.

These verses establish "seed-bearing plants" as healthy food. This includes grains, beans, legumes, nuts, seeds, vegetables, fruits, herbs, and spices. The variety of good foods is vast. However, God in his wisdom goes beyond this and adds to the smorgasbord. Look at Genesis 9:2–4: "All the animals of the earth, all the birds of the sky, all the small animals that scurry along the ground, and all the fish in the sea will look on you with fear and terror. I have placed them in your power. I have given them to you for food, just as I have given you grain and vegetables. But you must never eat any meat that still has the lifeblood in it." God is giving instructions to Noah about how to live after the flood.

Ezekiel 4:9 says, "Now go and get some wheat, barley, beans, lentils, millet, and emmer wheat, and mix them together in a storage jar. Use them to make bread for yourself during the 390 days you will be lying on your side."

This "Ezekiel Bread" has eighteen amino acids. Made from freshly sprouted organically grown grains, it's naturally flavorful and rich in protein, vitamins, minerals, and natural fiber with no added fat.

In Genesis, when God is talking about grains and seed-bearing plants, the translations are consistent in saying you *shall* eat these substances. This is in the form of a command, a directive. Yet in Deuteronomy, when referring to the use of animals as food, the wording is distinctly different.

As Dr. Rex Russell observes, time and time again the term *may* is used. This is done for a reason. God intended the use of seed-bearing plants and fruits as the foundation for healthy diets. However, he allows us to choose certain meats to supplement our diet.

Clean and Unclean

God emphatically and repeatedly states that it is permissible to eat clean animals and forbidden to consume the unclean. What is the difference?

If you refer back to the laws in Deuteronomy, the only clean animals are those that have divided hooves and chew the cud. It is no surprise that the only animals that fit both categories are the animals that consume vegetarian diets themselves! The scavengers and flesh eaters are considered unclean. According to scholars, a clean animal is defined by what it eats and the cleanliness of its digestive tract. (See Table 10 for a list of clean and unclean animals.) By avoiding the animals that consumed other animals, people avoided many of the diseases that were transmitted by the likes of parasites and worms. The group of unclean animals are omnivores because they literally will eat anything. What they eat, in turn, will be reflected in what you eat.

TABLE 10: CLEAN AND UNCLEAN ANIMALS

Clean Animals	Unclean Animals
Calf	Clams
Deer	Catfish
Goat	Shrimp
Ox	Pigs
Sheep	Rabbit
Chicken	Ostrich
Duck	Squirrel
Turkey	Crabs
Cod	Oyster
Flounder	Opossum
Halibut	Lobster
Salmon	Tuna

Does this distinction apply in today's world of strict manufacturing standards and quality control? Absolutely! The benefit in excluding the "unclean" animals today is not derived from the standpoint of communicable disease but from the avoidance of the consequences of high saturated fat diets. A quick perusal of the unclean animals shows a disproportionate number of them are meats high in saturated fat and cholesterol.

It is important to keep this designation in perspective. Abiding by these dietary laws does not imply any greater degree of spiritual attainment; all they refer to is the physical well-being of those who practice these habits. You don't achieve spiritual cleanliness by conforming to certain dietary restrictions. Old Testament dietary laws are not a way to earn entry into the kingdom of heaven, but they are a way to keep us healthy along the path. The occasional lobster, shrimp, or pork chop is fine since we're no longer under the law; just remember to maintain balance.

Listen and Obey

Examine Exodus 15:26: "If you will listen carefully to the voice of the Lord your God and do what is right in his sight, obeying his commands and keeping all his decrees, then I will not make you suffer any of the diseases I sent on the Egyptians; for I am the Lord who heals you."

Notice that this promise is conditional. You must first *listen* to the instructions that God has given to you, and then you must *follow* them! If you do those two things, then God has promised that you will not suffer any of the diseases of the Egyptians. What does this mean in today's world? You may be saying, "I don't have any Egyptian diseases, and I don't plan on having any!"

If you examine the Egyptian culture at the time of the Hebrew exodus, it is easy to understand the context and relevance of this verse. The Egyptians of this era had begun to fundamentally change their diet from one that was grain-based to one that was meat-based. These were good and prosperous times. Meat was a luxury and a symbol of prosperity, so it was widely consumed by the wealthy during this era. As a result, many Egyptians, especially the wealthy, developed problems consummate with such a dietary shift. Ancient writings are full of references to symptoms that are easily traced to heart disease and clogged arteries.

The most compelling evidence is found in the well-preserved remains of mummies that actually show advanced plaque in their arteries.

The Old Testament dietary laws also served to separate the Jews from their surroundings. It gave them a distinct identity in the midst of diverse cultures. Even today we often associate certain ethnic groups with distinct dietary practices, some more healthy than others.

God says plainly that if you stick to the things he created as food, then you will not suffer the diseases of those who choose foolishly. Remember that the first sin was not murder or adultery; it was eating something that God said man should not eat!

FAT IS NOT WHERE IT IS AT

Excessive fat intake is associated with a multitude of health problems. Atherosclerotic heart disease, the leading killer of adults, is intimately linked to dietary fat intake. High LDL cholesterol, diabetes, stroke, and obesity are all increased by a diet high in saturated and trans-fats. It is common knowledge that one of the leading sources of saturated fats in the average diet is from meat and meat products. The logic is clear. If you reduce the intake of bad fats, you will inevitably reduce the likelihood of developing myriad debilitating diseases.

Some fat is good—in fact, necessary—for proper body functioning. The key is moderating your intake and being careful of the type of fat. It has never been easier to quantify fat intake. Virtually every food product packaged and sold has nutritional labels that clearly state the fat content and its corresponding components.

The fallacy is that we have been able to come to these conclusions only through the miracle of modern science and the high-tech advances in research. Leviticus 7:23–27 reads, "Give the following instructions to the people of Israel. You must never eat fat, whether from cattle, sheep, or goats. The fat of an animal found dead or torn to pieces by wild animals must never be eaten, though it may be used for any other purpose. Anyone who eats fat from an animal presented as a special gift to the Lord will be cut off from the community. No matter where you live, you must never consume the blood of any bird or animal. Anyone who consumes blood will be cut off from the community."

Fat is essential in our diets, just in the right amounts and types. Fats from nuts, legumes, seeds, fruits, and vegetables (primarily unsaturated fats) are important in proper nutrition. Substitute olive oil for corn and sunflower oil and avoid trans-fat laden processed foods.

God, the Great Designer, knew what was best for his creation long before the invention of cholesterol-measuring devices or cardiac stress tests!

THE HORN OF PLENTY

Substitute unsaturated (mono-unsaturated or polyunsaturated) fats for saturated fats whenever possible. These fats, if used in place of others, can lower your risk of heart disease by reducing the total and low-density lipoprotein (LDL) cholesterol levels in your blood. One type of polyunsaturated fat, omega-3 fatty acids, may be especially beneficial to your heart. Omega-3s appear to decrease the risk of coronary artery disease. They may also protect against irregular heartbeats and help lower blood pressure.

Christianity is a religion of abundance. We believe in a gracious and loving God. A healthy diet is not about restriction. God is clear about what is good fuel for our bodies, and the selections are vast. The Old Testament does not hold a monopoly on healthy nutrition, but where instruction is given, it makes sense to follow. The secret for you is to explore the enormous number of healthy choices that are available and choose wisely.

There is a tremendous variety and selection of food available that we know to be healthy. These foods are abundant and, when used properly, will provide the cornerstone of any healthy lifestyle. A word of caution about overdoing it: You can get fat by eating only the "right" foods. *Too much* of the good stuff is just as bad as overindulging in pork rinds and ice cream. Moderation and discipline pave the way to dietary success.

Another implied concept from Jewish dietary laws is that food was largely consumed in its natural, raw, uncooked state in centuries past. There is no caution in Scripture that cooking food is bad. Common sense says, especially when it comes to meat, cooking is a preferable method of preparation (my apologies to the sushi lovers). However, fruits, grains, vegetables, and seeds should be consumed in their natural state. We know that many of the problems associated with diets are not so much the foods themselves but the method of preparation. Lose the grease and eat it raw! A general rule of thumb is that it is always best to consume a food as close to its natural state as possible. Luckily, there are many more resources for organically grown vegetables today than there were in the past. It's more inconvenient, and often more expensive, yet the long-term benefits are undeniable.

Many foods play a significant role in minimizing specific problems associated with menopause. Soy and soy products contain phytoestrogens, or substances with estrogen-like activity, which can be effective in attacking symptoms alone or in combination with other therapies. Foods such as leafy green vegetables and sea plants contain a great deal of calcium, which is critical in the menopausal years. These dietary instructions apply not only to midlife but from the cradle to the grave. Practicing good nutrition is critical in midlife and can minimize and sometimes eliminate menopausal problems. (See chapter 7 on complementary approaches.)

SUMMARY

You are what you eat. God has said that a diet based largely on vegetables, fruits, and plants is healthy and fights disease. Your midlife and menopause is a time for change, and one positive change is to shift your diet to one that will not only reduce menopausal symptoms but also improve your overall state of health. Some clean meats are acceptable, but everything should be weighed in the scale of moderation. The petition "Teach your children well" certainly applies to your responsibility to instruct those who respect and depend on you for advice about foods. When it comes to diet, think abnormally!

ACTION CHALLENGE

Write down everything you eat—morning, noon, and night—for three days. Read the list at the week's end. After the shock wears off, identify areas of weakness. Do you tend to overdo it more at night or in the morning? Are McEasy lunches your downfall? This can be an enlightening (and frightening) exercise, yet it is the foundation for initiating healthy change. To gather more specific information on diet and exercise, run, don't walk, to your local bookstore and pick up a copy (or two) of my book *Fat-Proof Your Family*.

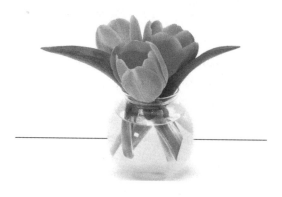

LOST LIBIDO: WHAT TO DO WHEN YOUR SEX DRIVE HAS DRIVEN OFF

Elisa was confused. She thought she was handling many of the changes of menopause effectively, yet she experienced one symptom that she couldn't get a grip on. She had no libido. Her sex drive had driven off, and she couldn't locate the map! It had not always been that way. She and her husband, Roy, had enjoyed a healthy sex life through most of their twenty-two years of marriage. Elisa was fifty-one and her periods had stopped seven months earlier. She had experienced a few hot flashes, but that was about it. When she came to see me she was concerned because this problem had begun to create friction in her marriage. We talked about her past sexual relationship and what was different now.

What became obvious after several minutes of discussion was that Elisa held many irrational thoughts and myths about sexuality in menopause. She had heard from her friends that it was natural to have a decreased libido as you age, and she believed this was normal. Her husband did not share this belief. She also thought that, as she aged, she was becoming less physically attractive to her husband. She had gained about six pounds over the past year, and she was embarrassed by the shift in her center of gravity. She reported that she had noticed some decreased lubrication during sex, but said she thought that was "par for the course." When questioned further, Elisa did admit that the few times she had sex over the past several months it had been physically uncomfortable.

The first step in solving Elisa's dilemma was to eliminate the myths and provide accurate information, essentially changing her attitude. Studies have shown some correlation between sex drive and age; however, you can have an active sex life well into your later years. One study in a national medical journal reports that women over fifty actually have fewer sexual problems than those under fifty.[1]

Next, Elisa and I explored the idea that sexual intimacy is much more than physical attractiveness. Her looks were changing, but her heart and soul were still what Roy loved. She knew this on a cognitive level but just needed to have it restated in the proper emotional context.

She initially didn't understand the link between aging, declining estrogen, and vaginal lubrication. Dryness in menopause arises from decreased secretion of the vaginal glands. This can lead to pain and discomfort with intercourse. Consciously or unconsciously, if it hurts, you don't want to do it! The good news is that there are solutions.

The resolution of Elisa's problem

> "Our sex drive naturally settles down after the raging hormones of youth, but never fades entirely as long as we stay healthy and fit. The brain is the number one sex organ, and beliefs determine our attitude to and experience of sex as in all else. To change our sex/love life, we need to change our thinking, and make quality time in our busy lives to nurture relationship and sex. It's never too late for love, romance, partnership, and a great sexual relationship."[2]

began with an attitude change. She began to understand the complex nature of the sex drive and discarded the belief that sex was not for the older generation. She changed the way she viewed her own sexuality and embraced the options available to her to counteract her physical problems. Some estrogen cream removed the pain and dryness she had experienced and restored her enjoyment without the fear of discomfort.

And, most important, she and Roy talked about the issue in an open and honest fashion.

THERE'S MORE TO LIBIDO THAN HORMONES

Sex drive, or libido, is one of the most complex of human behaviors. Some studies estimate that only a fraction of women actually suffer from hormone-induced decreased libido. In other words, there are few instances where a decreased sex drive is due solely to menopause. This may not be what you want to hear because you may be looking for a simple solution. Yet science supports the idea that hormones play a relatively small role in sex drive. Energy level, stress, marital discord, and past history all play a more significant role in determining libido. Since these are all individually unique experiences, it follows that sex drive is rarely the same for two people. Some medical problems such as diabetes and hypertension may interfere with libido. These maladies must be controlled before any realistic improvement in sexual functioning can occur. Be sure to take a list of all your medicines to your doctor and ask if any of them may affect sex drive. You may be surprised to find it is not that you are stressed or that your husband looks and acts like Big Foot—it may simply be your medications.

The signs of a low sex drive include:

- ✆ Less frequent sexual thoughts and fantasies

- ✆ Reduced sexual desire

- ✆ Reluctance to initiate sex

- ✆ Lack of desire for sex when you've gone without sex for days, weeks, or months (depending on what was previously normal for you).

In a survey, 35 percent of menopausal women said their sex life was actually better in menopause than before, whereas 25 percent said it was about the same.[3] However, there is no denying that there is a distinct role, albeit minimal, that hormones play in influencing sex drive.

I will never forget Margaret, a seventy-six-year-old firecracker, who was having difficulty remembering to take her hormones on time. I wanted to aid her in remembering, so I suggested that she associate taking her hormones with a common task she did automatically every day. I think I used the example of brushing her teeth or something similar.

She came back two months later and said, "Dr. Eaker, your suggestion worked beautifully. I haven't missed a pill. I simply take them after my husband and I make love."

My initial reaction was, *Oh no, she must have misunderstood me!* I explained to her that the pills were supposed to be taken every day.

She just smiled and said, "Yes, I know!" I learned my lesson that day. Never make assumptions about age and libido, as Elisa and I had.

PAINFUL INTERCOURSE

There certainly is a primary impact in that there is a connection between declining estrogen, progesterone, and testosterone and decreased libido. In addition, a secondary effect is that declining estrogen may lead to thinning of the vaginal and vulvar skin, which in turn leads to pain or discomfort with intercourse. Some women also note a decrease in response due to changes in the vulvar and vaginal tissues. The pain that some may experience with intercourse is likely the greatest inhibitor of sex drive.

> Up to 40% of postmenopausal women have symptoms of atrophic vaginitis.

Vaginal Estradiol

An obvious solution to dyspareunia (painful intercourse) is to replenish the vaginal tissues, increase lubrication, and stop the pain. Once this is accomplished, libido commonly improves. The most effective way of improving vaginal dryness and increasing lubrication is with the use of estradiol preparations. The scientific studies confirm this as the unquestionable leader in vaginal lining stimulation. The radical anti-estrogen crowd will just have to grin and bear this one, because the research shows that the complementary approaches to vaginal dryness are not as effective as topical estrogen.

Except for the occasional breast tenderness, the side effects of vaginal estrogens are minimal. There is very little absorption into the bloodstream, so the systemic risks are minimized. In fact, studies indicate that vaginal estrogen creams elicit minimal increases in blood estrogen levels. This effectively minimizes or eliminates many of the risks and side effects of oral estrogens. The estradiol preparations have an advantage for the vagina because they deliver the active ingredient directly to the tissues in need. Estradiol (bioidentical) can be applied as a cream or a vaginal tablet. An interesting product recently made available is a small flexible ring embedded with estradiol that fits in the vagina and gives a slow release of the hormone over several months. Some may like this because it eliminates the mess of the creams. Others might object to the idea of anything foreign staying in the vaginal canal for that length of time. It is a personal preference. Interestingly, many on oral hormone preparations often experience vaginal dryness and painful intercourse in spite of adequate doses. It is not uncommon to have to supplement with a vaginal estrogen, even while using a pill, shot, or patch.

Other Options

All is not lost for the purists who are die-hard estrogen haters; there are other options for improving vaginal lubrication and libido. Vitamin E gel or liquid has been shown to improve vaginal skin thickness and lubrication. You can take the 1,000 mg capsules and poke a hole in them and then rub the oil in the vaginal canal and on the labia twice a day. Remifemin, a standardized dose of black cohosh, has been effective in promoting normal lubrication.[4] There are several over-the-counter lubricants that have been helpful in treating this bothersome condition. They are non-hormonal and work with your body's own moisture to promote lubrication. Most pharmacies will carry several brands; just be aware that they are usually not as effective as topical estrogen, especially in severe cases or in women who have gone years past menopause.

Increasing the frequency of intercourse can actually improve vaginal dryness! Is God great or what? He has designed the body to work better if it is used more often. Now *that* is a nice piece of engineering! This knowledge is for women only. You don't have to share this news with your husband if you don't want to. Your secret is safe with me!

Don't forget to check the medicines you take. Antihistamines and diuretics (water pills) can dry the mucus membranes and the vaginal lining and should be avoided if possible. Also remember to increase your dietary intake of phytoestrogens (soy, legumes).

TESTOSTERONE

Now that we have conquered the vaginal problem (that sounds ominous, doesn't it?), let's look at some other ways to enhance libido. Testosterone has long been identified as the hormone that seems to exert a stimulating effect on sexual desire. This is especially apparent in those who have had their ovaries removed at the time of hysterectomy. Because the ovaries are your primary source of testosterone, and because they continue to produce testosterone during menopause, the use of testosterone is becoming more popular as a component of HT. Studies are conclusive that testosterone supplementation can enhance libido to a degree, and testosterone has also been credited with producing a general sense of well-being and energy in some women. Recent work also points out that the use of androgens (male hormones such as testosterone) in menopause may have a positive effect on lessening bone loss.[5]

Women produce small amounts of testosterone throughout their lives — about one-seventh the amount per day that men make. In women, testosterone is produced half in the ovaries and half in the adrenal glands. After menopause, testosterone production decreases gradually to two-thirds of premenopausal levels (unlike estrogen production, which decreases dramatically). In women who have had their ovaries removed, testosterone levels drop by half.

Testosterone is traditionally identified as the male hormone because it is produced in much higher quantities in men. When you hear of athletes using performance-enhancing drugs, this usually refers to a high dose of a form of testosterone. However, the ovary, that powerhouse of production, also makes testosterone. The adrenal glands, which sit on top of both kidneys, also produce testosterone and its precursors. So women do have testosterone flowing in their veins, albeit at a much lower level than men. Some women, however, actually produce an excess of testosterone and suffer from its effects: acne, oily skin, hair growth (where you don't want it), enlargement of the clitoris, and even deepening of the voice.

In those who still have their ovaries, testosterone continues to be produced after menopause, but the amounts can vary. Testosterone production falls dramatically if you have had your ovaries removed. Because of this dramatic drop of testosterone, you are more likely to suffer from decreased sex drive than someone who retains their functioning ovaries. Libido is a complex drive with many contributing factors. However, there is a legitimate place for replacing testosterone when it is low.

How do you know if it is low? The best test is the measurement of free or active testosterone in saliva or serum. This measures the active hormone in the system. Assessing testosterone levels can help clarify whether this is a significant player in libido problems. If you are symptomatic and your levels are low, then it is appropriate to consider testosterone replacement.

There are currently four common ways of administering testosterone. They mimic the methods of administering estrogen: pills, pellets, shots, and creams. Using the pure testosterone creams allows you to use a lower dose with fewer side effects. It also gives you more flexibility in dosing. A reasonable starting dose is a 5 mg/cc testosterone cream compounded by a pharmacy, with approximately a half of a cc rubbed on the abdomen or wrist once or twice a day. Levels can be monitored by saliva testing, but again you should rely largely on what you are experiencing to gauge success. Some may be experiencing decreased sensitivity or problems reaching orgasm. This may be helped by rubbing the testosterone cream directly on the clitoral area. This should be monitored for side effects such as enlargement of the clitoris. The testosterone cream can be used with or without estrogen. Monthly injections are used by some women, almost exclusively those who have had their ovaries surgically removed. Sub-dermal pellets containing testosterone, similar to those used to replace estrogen, can be implanted under the skin every four to six months. Finally, there are some patches that are being developed that provide a continual release of a low dose testosterone.

Side Effects

There are multiple studies that show the benefits of androgen (testosterone) replacement, but there are potential side effects. One of the most common and most disturbing side effects is increased hair growth, and I am not talking about on the head. Actually some women have reported hair loss from their heads! In various cases, some have had deepening of the voice, weight gain, enlargement of the clitoris, oily skin, and acne.

Probably the biggest potential concern with testosterone use is the effect on the blood lipids. Some studies suggest that testosterone increases the triglyceride levels and has a minimal effect on the total cholesterol (may be a slight decrease in HDL values). Recent work states that the addition of low-dose androgens to a standard HT regimen will not significantly decrease its effect on heart disease.[6] Studies are continuing, and the definitive word will be forthcoming. Testosterone cream produces lower blood levels than the oral testosterone and avoids some of the bothersome side effects. Once again, with the use of testosterone, either solely or in conjunction with other substances, you must look at the benefit: risk ratio. Make a decision based on your needs and in partnership with a knowledgeable health-care provider.

Some dim-witted, muscle-bound bodybuilders use very high dosages of testosterone, and the dangers from these are legion. The dosages used for testosterone replacement in women are vastly lower than those used by the Hulk wannabes, so if you use testosterone, you won't turn into an Arnold Schwarzenegger look-alike.

HERBAL REMEDIES

Many herbal products have been touted through the years as aphrodisiacs. Most of these are just fantasy and rely on the placebo effect for any benefit. This is another area where the hype is much greater than the reality. Most swindlers selling these products are actually selling hope in a quick fix, and it is virtually always a false hope.

Siberian ginseng, for example, has been long touted for its sexual enhancing ability. A search of the literature revealed only three studies that attempted to speak to this scientifically, and two of those were done on bulls! I can't recommend the use of ginseng in this capacity unless you own impotent bulls!

COMMUNICATION

Finally, one of the most important behaviors to practice for enhancing libido is developing effective communication with your husband. Talking about each other's sexuality, needs, wants, and problems can eliminate many misunderstandings. Some couples realize separately that there is a problem, yet they never discuss it. This in turn leads to many false assumptions that can fester like a boil and be quite damaging. These misperceptions can become like an insidious cancer that eats away at your relationship. You must bring up the issue if for no other reason than to acknowledge it exists. You may not perceive that there is a problem until your husband says there is!

> The word *aphrodisiac* comes from the Greek goddess of sensuality, Aphrodite. Medical science has not substantiated claims that any particular food increases sexual desire or performance.

What is not talked about can hurt you! It is not uncommon for sexual problems to go unaddressed simply due to a lack of understanding that a problem exists. That awareness can only come from one partner taking the initiative to say lovingly to their spouse that needs are not being met. Libido Avenue is a two-way street. You feed off the energy (or lack thereof) of your spouse. If they are suffering from a medical condition or a medicine effect that inhibits libido, it certainly affects you. Often it helps to go to your doctor's appointment as a couple and discuss the issue openly. It may be a safe forum to discuss feelings and needs in a directed, nonthreatening manner.

WHAT IS NORMAL?

Many couples struggle with knowing what is normal and what is not. Sexologists have debated this for years, and I suspect the debate will continue ad infinitum because this question is unanswerable.

Essentially, a normal libido is what is normal for you. What is your baseline? What feels right to you? How does Scripture instruct us on proper marital relations? Your answers to these questions impact your understanding of normal.

After a typical day of work, carpooling, household duties, homework, dinner, kid stuff, and laundry, very often the last thing on your mind is a romantic tryst. You just want to sleep, and rightly so. Many couples literally have to plan a date night to separate themselves from the routine hustle and bustle to even begin to think about sex. The expectations from TV, movies, and the print media are false, unrealistic, and damaging to couples. Thinking that your marriage is on the rocks because *Cosmopolitan* says that if you aren't having sex three times a week you are frigid, is just plain ludicrous. These so-called norms were propagated by such sham researchers as Alfred Kinsey and Shere Hite. The reality is that "normal" is determined by a variety of issues including morals, upbringing, genetics, and experience. Don't let some arbitrary number determine your sexual adequacy. Your standard should be Scripture, not the Kama Sutra.

Often, a change in libido is much more significant than someone who has always had a low sexual appetite. And remember that because God has made you different from your spouse, your individual sexual desires may vary tremendously. If that is the case, then your idea of normal is really based on your own experience and not the feelings of your partner. Determining what is normal for you as a couple takes some discussion and an honest evaluation of your differences. Then the task is to take these differences and blend them into the relationship in healthy ways that nourish both partners. Don't get caught in the trap of feeling you need some libido help without first going through this process. Rarely is decreased libido limited to just hormones. Even if testosterone is low, you must evaluate your stress level and lifestyle.

In solving a problem like poor sex drive, it is absolutely critical to involve your spouse. If sex drive is a problem in your relationship, talk about it openly with your spouse and support each other as you seek a solution. Some couples are greatly helped by seeing a trained counselor. The key is to find a person who is experienced in couples' therapy and comfortable with sexual issues. A healthy sexual relationship in the bounds of marriage is a God-ordained pleasure. Don't ignore this issue if either you or your husband perceives it to be a problem. Also, make sure there is compromise. As noted, rarely are two persons tuned the same.

Understand that this is compromise in the sense of meeting needs. This is not compromise when it comes to aberrant behavior or practices.

TREATMENT SUMMARY FOR DECREASED LIBIDO

1. Reduce stress and fatigue (two leading causes of decreased sex drive).
2. Explore relationship issues and discuss them with your husband. Sex is often a mirror of the health of the relationship.
3. Eliminate vaginal dryness with vitamin E, Remifemin, HT, vaginal inserts, and/or estrogen creams.
4. Use testosterone cream (5 mg/cc, ½ cc once or twice a day). If you are on HT, consider adding testosterone to the regimen (after an evaluation).

ACTION CHALLENGE

Once you have addressed and corrected any physical problems (vaginal dryness, pain, medicines) that may be playing a role, make a specific date night. Communicate with your husband your need for intimacy and romance, and enjoy the buildup to the evening. Commit to making this a regular event that takes priority.

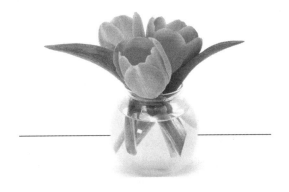

OSTEOPOROSIS: SKELETON SKILLS

Osteoporosis has the potential to be one of the most important words in your health vocabulary. The next time you are in church, look to your immediate left and look to your immediate right. You will see women at risk for osteoporosis because they are everywhere! Chances are good that you have some potential for thinning bones yourself. Women in menopause are especially at risk, thus the need for a discussion of osteoporosis in this book.

Osteoporosis means "porous bone." Call it brittle bones or thinning bones; it all means the same thing. It is a thinning of the material that makes the bones strong that may result in an increased risk for bone breaks. Osteoporosis is preventable; it can be identified early, and intervention can slow or stop its progression. The goal is to prevent the clinical result of the disease: fractures. Understand that no one ever died of osteoporosis. What you suffer from are complications of the disease, that is, the fractures and their subsequent effects.

Technological advances can now detect osteoporosis in its early stages, and this allows for aggressive and successful treatment. This is a critical development because, in most cases, osteoporosis arrives and progresses without symptoms. You don't know you have it until you fall and break a hip! In addition, we can accurately predict if you are at increased risk for developing osteoporosis. With this knowledge, you can take steps to make sure you are not one of the 250,000 who will suffer osteoporotic-related fractures next year.

BONES ARE ALIVE

Bone is a living, dynamic tissue. It is constantly being constructed and broken down throughout your life. The trabecular bone is the site for the majority of this activity. This is the internal part of the bone that gives it most of its strength and stability. When more bone is being broken down than is being built up, the net result is a weaker, less stable bone. Women are far more likely to be affected than men, especially after menopause. Estrogen stimulates the osteoblast (bone-building cells) and blocks the osteoclast (bone-eating cells). After menopause, when estrogen levels decline, the osteoblast are not as aggressive in building bone, and the osteoclast are hungrier and eat up more bone. The overall result is an acceleration of bone loss at menopause. This is significant because it is this loss of the trabecular bone in the hip, leg, and spine that leads to the increased risk for fractures a few years down the road.

There are many other factors that control bone loss, but for the sake of our discussion—and the fact that these other causes are relatively rare—I will limit this discussion to estrogen-deficiency-related osteoporosis. Some of the other causes are listed in Table 11.

Again, osteoporosis is the condition, and a fracture is a complication of the condition. You want to do everything you can to avoid developing osteoporosis, which in turn prevents pathological fractures.

TABLE 11: CLINICAL CAUSES OF OSTEOPOROSIS

Primary	
Menopause	
Aging (men and women)	
Secondary	
Renal failure	Hyperthyroidism
Intestinal bypass	Cushings syndrome
Malabsorption syndromes	Rheumatoid arthritis
Multiple myeloma	Anticonvulsants
Cancer	Antacids (chronic abuse)
Diabetes	Thyroid hormone therapy

STATISTICS

Should you be concerned about osteoporosis? Consider the statistics. Twenty-five million women are affected by osteoporosis. Over 250,000 women every year suffer a hip fracture directly or indirectly related to osteoporosis. If this number isn't frightening by itself, the long-term results of hip fractures are alarming. Up to 20 percent of women who fracture their hip die in the year after the break due to complications of the fracture. Of those who survive, almost 50 percent end up in a nursing home or an extended care facility. The medical economists estimate that hip fractures alone account for upwards of 10 billion dollars a year in health-care costs. Nearly 33 percent of women will fracture their hips in their lifetimes, and the greatest single risk factor is osteoporosis.[1] But remember, the good news is that this is a preventable disease!

The women at greatest risk of developing osteoporosis are thin, Caucasian, and inactive. The little old white lady who has Twinkies and Jack Daniels for breakfast, cigarettes for lunch, and watches soap operas all day will definitely have brittle

"Osteoporosis is a major public health threat for an estimated 44 million Americans, or 55% of the people 50 years of age and older. In the U.S., 10 million individuals are estimated to already have the disease and almost 34 million more are estimated to have low bone mass, placing them at increased risk for osteoporosis."[2]

bones (among other things). Not everyone develops osteoporosis, but as you can see from the following list, women in the menopausal age group have a greater likelihood of doing so.

If you are over fifty, you automatically fall into a high-risk category. Look at the list closely and identify how many risk factors you have. Notice that only a select few are unalterable, such as family history. (It really is a shame we can't pick our parents!) The vast majority of characteristics that place you in a high-risk category are behaviors and choices that you control.

— RISK FACTORS FOR OSTEOPOROSIS —

Caucasian

Oriental

Early menopause

Turner's syndrome

Small, thin frame

Poor diet

Excessive caffeine intake

High protein diet

Smoking

Physical inactivity

Excessive alcohol

Late puberty

Prior hysterectomy

Few or infrequent periods

Eating disorders (anorexia, bulimia)

Scoliosis

Family history

WHAT TO DO?

The prevention of osteoporosis should be the next great success story of public health education. The four A's pave the road to osteoporosis prevention.

Attitude

Take a proactive role in making decisions to alter behavior and lifestyle. Look again at the risk factors. What are the changes you can make beginning today that will minimize your potential for bone loss? Don't fall into the trap of procrastination. Studies are conclusive in showing that the earlier in life these healthy decisions are made, the less likely it is there will be trouble later on. The biggest obstacle in osteoporosis attitude adjustment is that people are not motivated to change. You don't have any outward or inward sign that this process is progressing. You feel fine. It's not like gaining weight, where the results are all too obvious. With osteoporosis, you often have no forewarning before it is late in the game. Now there are ways of detecting these changes very early, but the technology is still underutilized. (More about this later.) The ideal situation is to never need the technology. Change your attitude from the "head in the sand" mentality to one of prevention. Make up your mind that you are going to proactively maximize your bone-sparing ability.

Aptitude

Many women don't make the necessary lifestyle changes to prevent osteoporosis because they simply aren't aware of what changes to make. They don't know what behaviors make them more susceptible to bone loss. It's hard to be preventive when you don't know where to start. Learn all you can about different approaches to prevention, including medications, diet, and exercise. In today's information-overload world, there is no excuse for not knowing the facts of osteoporosis prevention and treatment. You are to be congratulated, as you are already taking the first steps by reading this book!

— LONG-TERM NEGATIVE CONSEQUENCES OF OSTEOPOROSIS —

Fractures

Dysfunctional and painful posture

Surgery

Loss of lung volume and breathing capacity

Disability

Poor endurance

Pain

Medical costs

Loss of strength

Hospital stays

Loss of height

Action

"More than 20 randomized, controlled trials suggest that regular physical exercise can reduce the risk of osteoporosis and delay the physiologic decrease of BMD. Short-term and long-term (measured up to 12 months) exercise training such as walking, jogging and stair climbing in healthy, sedentary postmenopausal women resulted in improved bone mineral content."[3]

Here we go again! Exercise, exercise, and more exercise. Weight-bearing exercise is a vital tool in preventing bone loss. Every study that has evaluated the relationship between exercise and osteoporosis has shown a strong protective benefit. Weight-bearing exercise strengthens bone and reduces its breakdown. This includes walking, running, aerobic exercising, weight lifting, dancing, using ski machines, and anything that puts strain on the bones. Swimming doesn't seem to provide much benefit because the water supports the bones. When bone has pressure applied to it through weight-bearing exercise, over an extended period of time, its density will increase. The pressure applied from muscle contractions, gravity, and the demands of exercise actually stimulates calcium deposition in the bone structure. The best thing you can do to strengthen your bones is to stay active.

Apothecary

There are several medications, herbs, foods, minerals, and vitamins that are important in the osteoporosis story. First, let's talk about diet.

DIET

Certain dietary excesses and deficiencies have been associated with increased bone loss. Luckily these are fairly rare for the average woman. Prevention can be as much about the avoidance of bad things as it is about consuming the right things. Unusual dietary habits that may promote osteoporosis include low calcium intake, high phosphorous intake, high-protein diets (a common weight-loss approach), excessive salt intake, and excess sugar consumption. All of these approaches can, over time, increase the metabolic loss of bone. This is not a rapid effect, so a week of high protein intake will not cause osteoporosis, but consistently eating excessive amounts of protein can increase the leeching of calcium from the bone leading to bone structure deterioration.

What is the highest source of phosphates in the average diet? Soft drinks! If you drink a six-pack of diet or regular cola a day (and you would be amazed how many do), you may be increasing your risk for brittle bones in the future. This will have a dramatic impact as the baby boomers age since they are the first generation that has consumed soft drinks in such mass quantities. Bone loss is cumulative, so the more you lose early on, the greater your risk later in life.

DO THE RIGHT THING

Enough of the negative! Let's focus on the proactive things you can embrace to reduce or possibly prevent osteoporosis. A vegetarian diet is associated with a lower risk of osteoporosis.[4] This may be due to the decreased protein intake in a vegetarian diet.

Green leafy vegetables are the major components of a vegetarian diet that aid in preventing bone loss. They serve as an important source of boron, calcium, and vitamin K. Vitamin K is essential to the proper mineralization of the bone, and deficiencies can increase the severity of bone fractures. Boron is an essential ingredient in the proper interaction of vitamin D and estrogen on the bone. The consumption of phytoestrogens (see chapter 7) may help in the overall battle against osteoporosis. Some of the isoflavonoids in plants are being investigated for their interaction with calcitonin, a hormone that regulates calcium metabolism.

Calcium tends to get the headlines, but several other vitamins and minerals are also important in proper bone health. Vitamin D helps to regulate how the kidneys excrete calcium. This in turn controls the blood level of calcium, which directly impacts the absorption rate from the bone. Vitamin D deficiency can be manifested in the older population who may not get much sun exposure, because sunlight causes a chemical change in the skin that forms vitamin D. Studies support the recommendation to consume at least 400 IU of vitamin D a day, either through diet or supplements.

Magnesium is also very important. Magnesium activates enzymes that help form new calcium crystals. It is also important in helping vitamin D convert to its active form and in helping with proper function of the bone-related hormones: parathyroid hormone and calcitonin. Women with severe osteoporosis have a lower magnesium level in their blood than women without osteoporosis.[5] A 1990 study looked at combining adequate calcium with magnesium and found this regimen not only decreased bone loss, but also increased the remineralization of weight-bearing bones.[6] Ingesting the proper ratio of magnesium and calcium is more effective than simply taking calcium. Research has suggested that the optimal magnesium intake is 400 to 800 mg per day.

Manganese, folic acid, strontium, vitamin B6, vitamin B12, and silicon have all been linked to good bone health. Most are critical components in the bone formation process. In reality, a good diet will provide plenty of each of these vitamins and minerals, so specific supplementation is not needed. Most good multivitamin formulations will contain adequate amounts of all of these.

CALCIUM

Ninety-nine percent of the body's calcium is stored in the bones and teeth.

Calcium is universally known as the crucial mineral in osteoporosis prevention. There is no question that calcium supplementation has been shown to reduce bone loss in postmenopausal women.[7] More important, calcium added to the diet has been shown to reduce the incidence of the dreaded consequence of osteoporosis: the fracture. Calcium is a major component of trabecular bone matrix, and without adequate amounts of calcium, the proper bone consistency cannot be maintained. The National Institute of Health and the National Academy of Sciences recommend 1,000 to 1,200 mg of calcium a day for women under sixty-five and 1,500 mg a day for those over sixty-five. These recommendations are based on years of research and data.[8] These represent total daily dietary intake amounts. The reality is that most standard American diets provide only about 500 to 800 mg of calcium a day. For those who don't consume dairy products or many vegetables, this value may be even less. It follows, then, that to get adequate calcium without a major change in your diet, you must supplement. Based on the data, a supplement with at least 500 mg of calcium is recommended. There is some evidence that the body cannot absorb any more than this at one time, and taking more than 500 to 600 mg a day is not helpful.

Calcium carbonate is one of the most readily available calcium supplements. It is the form of calcium in products such as Tums EX, Os-Cal, Viactiv, and Caltrate. Some argue that calcium citrate is better absorbed, yet research suggests that the true clinical value of this increased absorption is negligible. The most important factor is tolerability. Some calcium products irritate the gastrointestinal tract, causing stomach upset or constipation. Trial and error is the best method to determine which calcium supplement is right for you.

Another advantage of refined calcium carbonate is its low lead content. Calcium derived from oyster shells, dolomite, or bone meal may contain undesirable amounts of lead that could negatively impact your health if taken over a long period of time. Other good sources of calcium are those combined with citrate, gluconate, or fumerate. Read the labels. It will say specifically on the label what type of calcium and what amount it contains. If a tablet form of calcium seems to irritate your stomach, try a liquid-based calcium supplement like Citracal. When purchasing calcium supplements, be sure to look for the *elemental calcium* content, not the total content. For instance, a pill containing 500 mg of calcium carbonate provides 200 mg of elemental calcium. Calcium citrate usually provides less *elemental calcium* per pill; therefore, you may need to take relatively more numbers of pills per day depending on your needs. Most calcium supplements will list the elemental calcium content on their packages. If it isn't listed, the simplest way to determine how much elemental calcium is in a supplement is to look at the Nutrition Facts label. For calcium, the Percent Daily Value (% DV) is based on 1,000 mg of elemental calcium, so every 10 percent in the Daily Value column represents 100 mg of elemental calcium (0.10 x 1,000 mg = 100 mg). For example, if a calcium supplement has 60 percent of the Daily Value, it contains 600 mg of elemental calcium (0.60 x 1,000 mg = 600 mg).[9]

PARADE OF STARS

Calcium-Rich Foods

Milk (skim, low-fat, or whole)

Plain yogurt

Frozen yogurt with fruit

Ricotta cheese

Sardines

Cooked greens (collards or mustard)

Firm cheeses (swiss, edam, brick, cheddar, gouda, colby, mozzarella)

Calcium-fortified orange juice

Several medications have an impact on preventing and treating osteoporosis: estrogen, progesterone, biphosphonates, SERMs, and calcitonin.

The studies are voluminous and conclusive that taking estrogen reduces bone loss. Even the most radical critics agree that estrogen loss at menopause accelerates overall bone loss, and the use of estrogen can slow the process.[10] Is estrogen use the only way to prevent osteoporosis? Will you become a humpbacked, creaky old lady if you don't use estrogen (as some of the drug companies subtly imply)? Absolutely not!

There are options. Can estrogen be an important part of osteoporosis prevention and treatment? You bet it can! It is all about balance. Are you at high risk for osteoporosis? Are you doing the right things with your diet and exercise? Can the advantages of HT override the risks for your individual situation? These are the kind of questions that must be answered when considering a medication like estrogen. For many, this is most efficiently done in consultation with a doctor who is well-versed on options. Remember what I said earlier, however: Never take estrogen solely for bone health.

With knowledge as a foundation, ask your doctor about diet, herbs, vitamins, and other medications to help prevent osteoporosis. If you do choose to go with HT, focus on utilizing a form of estradiol. Tri-est, estriol, and creams have not been effective at preventing fractures. Don't gamble on these unproven medicines if you are at high risk for osteoporosis.

The role of progesterone in bone physiology is not clear. There are progesterone receptors on the osteoblast (bone-builders), yet the exact effect of progesterone on these cells has not been determined. In laboratory experiments, progesterone has been shown to promote bone growth in animals, but this has not convincingly been shown in humans. In women who have a known progesterone deficiency (anovulatory), there is a measurable increase in the rate of bone loss when compared to women with normal blood progesterone levels. This provides presumptive evidence that progesterone is linked to bone metabolism. What is lacking is a long-term study of natural progesterone replacement (comparing bone loss or gain to a placebo), and then a follow-up of these patients for several years to see if there is an actual decrease in the fracture incidence. There is some data that suggests the addition of natural progesterone to estrogen regimens enhances the overall bone-sparing ability, but this is with very small numbers of subjects.

Dr. John Lee, in his book *What Your Doctor May Not Tell You About Menopause*, claims that natural progesterone cream not only slows bone loss but also actually builds bone. This is a premature conclusion, and the data just doesn't support using progesterone cream as a way to prevent bone loss. The data he uses to support this hypothesis is flawed, and therefore his conclusions are unreliable. Several of the studies he quotes to support his arguments are from work done on micronized progesterone, an oral form that differs in absorption from the cream. These studies had very small numbers of participants, and it is invalid to take those results and assume the same would apply to the cream.

Dr. Jerilynn Prior of the University of British Columbia has done a great deal of research on bone and menstrual cycle irregularity in athletes. Lee and others often quote her as a source of evidence for the use of progesterone in osteoporosis prevention. However, her work, if you actually read the studies, is on a very specific population and is largely observational. Natural progesterone cream has not been tested as to its long-term effect on osteoporosis by her or anyone else.

Natural progesterone cream has many useful applications; however, using it as your sole aid against osteoporosis is wrong and dangerous.

Alendronate (Fosamax), Risedronate (Actonel), and Ibandronate (Boniva) are drugs known as biphosphonates that are approved by the FDA for the prevention and treatment of post-menopausal osteoporosis. They work directly on the bone to prevent bone breakdown by blocking the action of the osteoclasts (bone-eaters). Their only benefit is on the bone, and they will do nothing to counteract any of the other symptoms of menopause. Their long-term safety has yet to be determined, although short-term safety has been well documented. There is some concern about a rare complication of bone breakdown in the jaws of those using these medications; however, this complication was noted in very select patients with underlying medical problems and not found in healthy folks.

Some have complained about digestive discomfort and esophagitis (reflux) with the biphosphonate medicines. Anything that interferes with convenience lessens compliance. Once-a-week and once-a-month formulations of these medicines are now available that reduce these side effects and improve compliance. You can expect other biphosphonates on the market in years to come, including injectable and intravenous preparations. This is a huge market for the drug companies, and the competition is fierce. Once again, it becomes an individual decision as to whether the advantages outweigh the disadvantages for your situation.

Calcitonin is a hormone produced by the thyroid gland that is responsible for calcium use in the bone. It is approved by the FDA for treatment—not prevention—of osteoporosis, so it should only be considered in patients with already diagnosed osteoporosis. Calcitonin actually increases bone density and may reduce bone pain from fractures and osteoporotic changes, and it is given by injection or a nasal spray. In the short term it is a safe medication, but again, the long-term studies of safety are lacking.

Raloxifene (Evista) is one of a new class of medications called the SERMs. This stands for selective estrogen receptor modulators. They have been nicknamed "designer estrogens" by the media. What that means in real English is that these drugs selectively attach to certain receptors and avoid other similar receptors. In the case of Raloxifene, it stimulates the estrogen receptors in the bone but not in the uterus. In the breast it actually appears to act as an anti-estrogen. In fact, when this drug was first tested, it was being evaluated as a possible treatment for breast cancer. The beneficial effects on bone were first noted as a welcomed side effect; however, as the research developed, it was found that the bone benefit was truly remarkable and marketable. Even though it is a hormone with some estrogen-like effects, it will not counteract any of your menopausal symptoms. In fact, a number of women using Raloxifene experience hot flashes. Women with a uterus can use this safely, as there is no effect or increased risk for uterine overgrowth, bleeding, or cancer.

At the time of this writing, researchers have been following patients on Raloxifene for several years and have seen a significant reduction in the occurrence of breast cancer in users as compared to the general population. This data is preliminary but encouraging. We may soon have a medication that will help osteoporosis and possibly reduce the incidence of breast cancer. Another potential benefit of Raloxifene is that there appears to be a lowering of total cholesterol in users as compared to the general population. Whether this will have a clinical effect on the reduction of heart disease remains to be seen.

Another category of osteoporosis medicines combines both an anti-resorptive and a stimulatory effect on the bone. In other words, they help build bone and block its loss. Teriparatide (Forteo) is an example of this type of medicine, and its major drawback is that it must be given as a daily subcutaneous injection, much like insulin for diabetics.

These are some of the currently available medicines for the prevention and treatment of osteoporosis, but expect more soon, as this is a hot area for research.

MEDICATIONS—WHO NEEDS THEM?

Who should consider using these medications? Anyone who is in a high-risk position! And that means almost all women in menopause. Hear what I said: *Consider* using something. Look at your options. Should everyone use these medications? Absolutely not! These medicines are only to be considered after making the proper lifestyle changes, dietary modifications, and exercise. Part of the decision-making process is to consider whether osteoporosis or osteopenia (the mild loss that proceeds osteoporosis) already exists, and estimate your risks for it progressing.

Technology exists to identify osteoporosis in its early stages. The most accurate and common measurement is known as bone densiometry. You may hear it referred to as BMD or bone mineral densiometry. This technique uses X-ray technology and computer calculations to assess the density or mass of individual bones or of the entire body. The gold standard in BMD measurement is the DEXA, or dual-energy X-ray absorptiometry, because of its precision and accuracy. The most common areas tested are the lumbar spine and the hip, mainly because these are the two areas most profoundly affected by osteoporosis.

The National Osteoporosis Foundation has published guidelines as to who should have BMD measurements. These are found in Table 12. In general, anyone who is considering using a medication to prevent osteoporosis, has a strong family history of the disease, or has two or more high risk factors should have a bone densiometry. Whether or not you need a bone densiometry is dependent on your own medical situation and your risk factors.

Table 12: Bone Densiometry Guidelines

- All postmenopausal women under 65 who have one or more additional risk factors

- All women 65 and over.

- Postmenopausal women who present with fractures.

- Women who are considering therapy for osteoporosis, if BMD would facilitate the decision.

- Women who have been on hormone replacement therapy for five years or more.

Other cheaper and simpler methods of detecting bone loss are available; however, they suffer from a lack of accuracy and specificity. The heel ultrasound is a small office-based machine that measures differences in the bone's reflection of sound waves and has been shown to be accurate in predicting fracture risk. It is only a screening device in that abnormal results should be followed with a full BMD to determine if and where osteoporosis is present. Ultrasound is easy to do, painless, and inexpensive, so it functions well as a first approach to screening for some women. It is less sensitive; so it should not be the determining factor regulating treatment. Because change in the bone is slow, these screenings should be done no more often than every two years to give meaningful serial data.

Two other bone-related tests you should be familiar with are measures of bone loss and bone formation. These are most useful in following the effectiveness of therapy. They cannot be used by themselves to make a diagnosis of osteoporosis. If you are taking a medication and are curious about whether it is working, you can opt for one of these approaches. The bone-loss test checks the urine for bone breakdown products, while the bone-buildup evaluation is a blood test that looks at the by-product of bone production. Both are fairly accurate. They can be useful in assessing whether a certain regimen is working, which may contribute to the decision to continue your present treatment or change directions.

ACTION CHALLENGE

Prevention of Osteoporosis

1. Identify and minimize risk factors.
2. Consider bone densiometry.
3. Eat a vegetarian diet.
4. Exercise (weight-bearing).
5. Get adequate elemental calcium (500–800 mg/day), magnesium (400–800 mg/day), and boron (3–5 mg/day).
6. Consider HT, SERM or a biphosphonate if high-risk.
7. Follow effectiveness with urine or blood tests.

Treatment of Osteoporosis

1. Have a DEXA bone mineral density test.
2. Use an osteoporosis treatment medication (ET, biphosphonate, SERM, etc.).
3. Follow all the prevention suggestions.

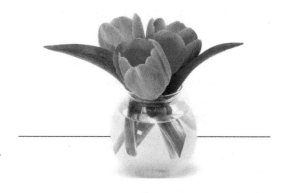

THE HEALING POWER
OF PRAYER

You may come to the menopausal years mature in body, mind, and spirit. This accumulated wisdom and life experience can be a joy and a burden. There is joy in knowing that wisdom comes from experience and action, both of which can be yours in this transition. However, there is fear in change, especially when it is unexpected or uninvited. Menopause is change, and a great deal of this book has been devoted to how to adapt to this change both physically and emotionally, yet one thing is still lacking. To complete the triad of wellness (mind, body, and spirit), we must explore the component of spirituality. Obviously this realm is vast, so I have chosen to focus on one aspect of a Christian worldview that has a direct impact on menopause—that of prayer and healing. Aging increases our risk for a variety of physical and emotional ailments. Your worldview, encompassing such things as the healing power of prayer and God's response to your physical and emotional ills, contributes to your coping with and understanding of illness. I have worked with a number of women over the years who have found the strength and courage to face transitional challenges through their faith. Let's look specifically at the relationship between faith, medical science, and menopause.

God heals! Whether it is PMS, menopause, or cancer, your physical health and mental well-being are intimately linked to your spiritual health. This is not meant to imply that the only way to physical health is through supernatural healing. Don't misunderstand. There are many physically and mentally healthy individuals who have no interest in their spiritual development. However, to achieve lasting, true, joyous well-being and balance, the spirit—that part of you that makes you human—can't be excluded. Daily prayer can be as vital to a healthy midlife experience as exercise, herbs, and diet. Open your mind and heart to the possibility that prayer can be a powerful conduit for healing and an essential part of health. Prayer is the thread that is woven throughout the tapestry of midlife, giving it strength and unity.

For many, the association of prayer and healing is a natural one. You may have grown up in a tradition where the connection between your physical health and your religious beliefs was encouraged and supported. Many churches embrace healing ministries and parish nurse programs. For others, the correlation between prayer and healing may be weak or even unrecognized. You may identify prayer and healing with a self-righteous, leisure-suited television evangelist touching the screen

There was a time about 15 years ago when those who were actively investigating the linkages between religion and health could have fit around a single conference table. A very small one. Today, the epidemiology of religion and the larger field of clinical research on religion and spirituality are well established in the scientific world and in the public consciousness. The U.S. National Institutes of Health has convened invited conferences, established expert working groups, and funded considerable empirical research in this area.[1]

and yelling, "Be gone, you evil hot-flash demon!" That is a sad but true caricature of healing prayer and not the focus of this chapter. I am concerned with a revitalization of the idea of unity of mind, body, and spirit.

PRAYER AS A DAILY PRACTICE

Consider prayer as a daily discipline for healthy living. Just as you would get up in the morning and brush your teeth (or soak your dentures) and reach for the vitamins, so you could (and should) have prayer as a part of your daily regimen. This is not meant to equate prayer and dental hygiene, but to illustrate how contemplation and talking with God should be a daily, common practice.

For a long time I, like many others, thought of the relationship of prayer and healing from a last-resort mentality: When all else fails, pray. Prayer was the fail-safe, Hail Mary attempt to pull it out at the end. I lived under this falsehood for the first few years of my medical practice. I would pray for folks when I believed nothing else (medical therapeutics or surgery) could alter the outcome. Scripture teaches that this is only a superficial understanding of what prayer is. This utilization of prayer places it on par with the lottery. The reality is that prayer is essential, helpful, and comforting even when you are not in a crisis. Certainly there is a place for intercessory prayer in desperate situations, yet connecting daily with God provides a perpetual healing salve to the spirit. Don't wait until you are sick to utilize this wonderful and powerful gift. Prayer is more than a tool; it is a sacred privilege. God heals through his grace and wisdom, and prayer has an impact. Effective healing prayer begins with a humble and repentant spirit that is more concerned with knowing God than healing. Praying or going to church only in order to get healed—external religiosity—is ineffective, inauthentic, and unworthy.

Begin to see prayer as a vital, daily part of your quest for health.

THREE MODELS OF HEALING

A while ago my younger brother Bruce drove himself to the hospital with a severely infected appendix. At the time, Bruce had four children, all under the age of six. As you can imagine, there was no getting this crowd up and dressed at four in the morning for something as silly as a ruptured appendix. So his wife stayed home with the kids, and he ended up driving solo to surgery.

As I was thinking about him the next day, it occurred to me that during his hospitalization and recovery, he would deal with three distinct yet interrelated modes of healing.

The first, and by far the most immediate, is the mechanical mode of healing. This is surgery to remove the infected tissue. No intelligent person would disagree that this is a necessary and helpful tool in this situation. As young surgeons in training, we are taught, "When in doubt, cut it out!" Before surgery and anesthesia were rendered relatively safe, many died from rupture of the appendix and subsequent sepsis. So utilizing the mechanical healing model is highly effective and desirable in this scenario.

"Each year nearly 700,000 patients present to the ER with suspected appendicitis; about half of these patients will have atypical or equivocal signs and symptoms. Thirty percent of all appendicitis patients have a perforated appendix, which can be fatal in 5% of cases."[2]

The second mode of healing is mind-body healing, the mental mode. This is healing that is influenced by how we think, feel, and believe. Unfortunately, many Christians have incorrectly associated this type of healing with various New Age philosophies, so they have an unfounded bias against the legitimacy of this healing tool. God designed this relationship between mind and body as part of his perfect plan for our healthy existence. We are much more than our physical bodies. For example, how you feel about an illness can dramatically affect its course. There is a new branch of science called psychoneuroimmunology that studies how thoughts and emotions impact your immune system. It has been scientifically proven that emotions such as anxiety and anger can actually decrease the function of white blood cells, your body's defense against disease. So how stressed Bruce is, how much faith he has in his surgeon, and his belief about his own state of health can all impact his healing.

The third mode of healing that I envision for Bruce is the healing power of prayer, the spiritual mode. To date this has not been as scientifically validated as the first two modes (as it will not need to be), yet I firmly believe its role is just as powerful and effective as the other two. Prayer has long been associated with healing, and it is only recently that this unnatural separation has developed. For thousands of years the healer in a community was often also the religious leader. There was an acknowledgment of the dualistic nature of health: physical and spiritual. With the advent of the Enlightenment and the age of reason, science began to separate from faith. Science measured the observable and faith dealt with the unobservable. Through the years this chasm has widened to the point that, for many, there is an impenetrable demarcation separating science and religion. This is unfortunate (and unnecessary), but there are signs of change on the horizon.

These three approaches—biomechanical, mind-body, and spirit—are not exclusive to one another. They work best to achieve healing when they work together. The wise person is the one who doesn't focus on only one mode but embraces all the gifts and graces that are given so freely. It is impossible to be totally healed without some influence from each area: the biomechanical, the mental, and the spiritual.

MY BIAS

Before we progress too far into this discussion, I feel compelled to outline my bias. Everything you read is presented through the often myopic lens of my worldview, and this naturally influences the presentation of even objective facts. I am a Christian (big surprise there), and I believe in an omniscient, omnipotent, loving, and healing God. John Wesley, the father of Methodism, wrote extensively about healing, the use of natural remedies, and the power of healing prayer. Wesley's treatises on the importance of healing the whole person, physically and spiritually, have influenced many, including myself. So I am initiating this discussion based on the firm belief that prayer is a wonderfully miraculous force for healing.

I am a physician, and as such I was trained to be analytical and logical in my approach to healing. I was taught that "first do no harm" meant don't subject a patient to any therapy that is either unproven or more hazardous than its potential benefit. You expect your health-care provider to suggest treatments that are effective, practical, and safe. Leaps of faith should be used sparingly in medicine, because if you leap indiscriminately you can land in some deep holes. It is with this background, a strong belief in a healing God, and a devotion to the scientific method, that I want to consider the relationship between religion and health.

DEFINITIONS

Healing refers to much more than just ridding the body of disease. The origin of the word *heal* is *haelan,* which means to make whole. Whole in this sense is the equilibrium among mind, body, and spirit. This is the healing triad where each component is dependent on the other, and, to achieve balance, all parts must be in harmony. It is like a three-legged stool, where all the legs must be balanced or the stool teeters and totters. In this concept, *health* is defined as achieving a balance of all three components. Simply getting rid of a sore throat with an antibiotic is curing, and that is a good thing; however, healing involves going beyond the bacteria and exploring causes such as diet, stress, relationships, and spiritual well-being, all of which may play a role in initiating, perpetuating, or healing that sore throat.

I am not a theologian. I aspire to the KISS philosophy: Keep It Simple . . . and Scriptural. My definition of prayer is simple: communication with God. Prayer can take many different forms. Many would assume that it is talking out loud in English to a patriarchal male with a long, flowing beard somewhere in the sky. That image and approach is okay, but this communication can be many other things. It can be songs, music, dance, or meditative silence. It can be anytime you and God are together, and that is all the time! This is the essence of what Paul meant when he entreated the Ephesians to "pray in the Spirit at all times and on every occasion. Stay alert and be persistent in your prayers for all believers everywhere" (Ephesians 6:18).

I am not normal. You see, I run marathons for fun! When I run, often I pray. As I lope along the riverbank and the fog creeps down the river and the sun gushes over the crown of the trees, I feel very close to God. It's like when the psalmist bathes in the glory of creation as the fingerprints of God. The physical experience of running in God's beauty is overwhelming. I have had some real heart-to-heart talks with God on those long runs. Granted, at times I am praying, "God, please let me make it back before I die of exhaustion!" But for the most part, it is a joyful time alone with the Creator in which I am renewed and refreshed.

Prayer is a dialogue. It is two-way communication. If you spend all of your time talking, how will you ever hear answers to your prayers?

Think about constructing a relationship with your spouse. If you spent all your time talking and never listening, you wouldn't know him at all. So it is with God. How can you expect to strengthen a relationship unless you hear him? Be still, be quiet, and be open.

When my daughter was about five years old, I was attempting to teach her about prayer. I creatively used the analogy that prayer is like a long-distance phone call to God. This seemed to click with her. A few nights later when we were saying her prayers, she looked up and said, "Daddy, I know why we always pray at night."

"Why is that, darling?" I asked.

She replied, "That's when the rates are cheapest!"

PRAYER IN THE WORKPLACE

As a physician who promotes healing on a daily basis, I am intrigued with the idea of incorporating prayer into my medical practice. Believing as I do, I *have* to incorporate prayer into my practice to be consistent with my values. I must pray for and with my patients. I understand that patients come to me as a physician first and foremost, yet I can't ignore my calling to be a witness for Christ. If I ignored that testimony, would it be tantamount to spiritual malpractice? This is an area of great controversy and debate in the medical profession. I agree with some critics that proselytizing in the office may not be appropriate given the dynamics of the doctor-patient relationship; however, since a patient's spiritual beliefs may impact their health, it is imperative and appropriate for me to understand and inquire about those beliefs. Taking a spiritual history is often equally as important as the physical exam. Understand that my role as a physician is not limited to Christian patients. There is a virtual smorgasbord of religions practiced

The first study of physicians' religious beliefs has found that 76% of doctors believe in God, and 59% believe in some sort of afterlife. The survey, performed by researchers at the University of Chicago and published in the July 2005 issue of the Journal of General Internal Medicine, found that 90% of doctors in the United States attend religious services at least occasionally, compared to 81% of all adults. Fifty-five percent of doctors say their religious beliefs influence how they practice medicine.

by patients I care for. Their religious practices impact their health just as much as a Christian's beliefs impact theirs.

This understanding has been a transformational journey for me. For years it was as if I would walk into my office and put God on the coatrack and then pick him up again at the end of the day. I was living on two parallel tracks—my job and my religion—and each was aware of the other, yet they never seemed to interact. Many of you may be living this same dichotomy. The dissonance eventually forced me to find some way of merging the secular and the spiritual. If I was to be consistent to both the science and the faith, I had to successfully integrate the two without compromising either. In order to merge these seemingly divergent beliefs into a lifestyle, I began to ask questions.

> "A librarian was fired for wearing a cross necklace to work. A federal court declared the library policy unconstitutional and said it violated the Free Speech and Free Exercise Clauses of the First Amendment. 'This is a very important decision that underscores the fact that employees have constitutional rights to express their faith in the workplace so long as that expression does not interfere with the work setting,' said Frank Manion, Senior Counsel of the American Center for Law and Justice, which represents the library employee. 'The fact that our client was fired for wearing a cross pendant on a necklace to work is not only absurd but unconstitutional as well. This decision sends an important message that employers cannot discriminate against employees who choose to express their religious beliefs in the workplace.'"[3]

Are prayer and science compatible? Can they coexist or are they mutually exclusive? Can prayer be tested? What is the evidence that prayer is effective? Is this an issue solely of faith, or can science demonstrate its effectiveness?

The God of the universe is not threatened or intimidated by questions; he encourages them because the answers you seek are based in truth. All truth is of God, so if we seek the truth (and that is the goal of science), we are seeking to better know God. We know by faith that prayer heals. Is this to be left to the realm of the mystic, or are we to utilize God-given techniques to bolster our faith?

CAN PRAYER BE TESTED?

This begs the question, Is employing the scientific method appropriate to validate this miraculous ability? This is not about proving or disproving prayer. (I have trouble doing long division; therefore, I'm not about to try to fully understand the mystery of prayer.) It is about demonstrating the awesome power and grace of the Creator in providing this glorious tool for us to employ. Faith does not lend itself easily to scientific scrutiny, nor should it. By definition, faith involves unproven (by logic) and unseen beliefs. Dr. Larry Dossey, a Texas internist who has written extensively on the healing power of prayer, said, "When we test prayer we are not storming heaven's gates. These studies can be sacred reverent exercises. Testing prayer can actually be a form of worship, a ritual in which we express our gratitude for this remarkable phenomenon."[4]

I know by faith that prayer is answered; can science confirm that? Understand that science, by its nature, cannot conclusively prove or disprove faith issues. You may ask, "If faith is independent of science, then why bother?" It is worth analysis for many reasons, but one important consequence is its evangelistic application. There are many people who speak the language of science who would never open the door to the Gospel unless it was presented in terms they could understand. A missionary in Japan would not be very effective unless she spoke Japanese. These studies allow the Good News to be presented in a way that is understood by many from scientific, skeptical, or secular backgrounds.

The person suffering from chronic pelvic pain is a patient whom most gynecologists dread, mainly because the origin of the pain is both difficult to identify and troublesome to treat. A competent physician starts with the assumption that the pain really exists. Trouble often arises when readily available techniques fail to elicit a pain etiology. At times I have found myself in this situation, thinking, *Well, if I can't identify the pain source, then the pain must be in her head.* But that's not the case—I just can't explain it given my current knowledge and technology. The same applies to prayer. We know prayer works by our faith. If science validates that, good for science. If it falls short, the problem is with science, not faith.

If we are going to study prayer, how are we going to define it? How do you measure prayer? What is a good outcome and what is not? These and other issues must be critically evaluated by anyone attempting to assess the scientific evidence for prayer. This is not bringing God into the laboratory; it is bringing the laboratory to God. It is not a simple, straightforward exercise, but one with many twists and turns that can derail even the best research design.

PRAYER STUDIES

To answer these questions, I did what physicians commonly do: I began a search of the medical literature. I was astounded by what I discovered. The volume of literature on the healing power of prayer in legitimate scientific journals is astonishing. One recent volume, *The Handbook of Religion and Health* by Harold Koenig, lists over five hundred studies evaluating the association between religion and mental and physical well-being.

One of the first and most interesting studies was published by the *Southern Medical Journal* in 1989 by a cardiologist in San Francisco named Dr. Randolph Byrd. He randomly assigned 393 patients admitted to the coronary care unit of a local hospital to be in either a "prayed-for" group or a "non-prayed-for" group. These were very sick people; their admitting diagnosis was either a heart attack or a presumed heart attack. Neither the patients nor the doctors or nurses knew who was in each group, so this was a randomized, double-blind study. The groups doing the praying were given the first names of the patients, their diagnosis, and their condition. The prayer groups were told to pray for each patient to have a rapid recovery with few complications. It was interesting to note that the prayer groups were in San Francisco as well as other parts of the state.

The results were exciting. The "prayed-for" group was five times less likely to need antibiotics during their hospitalization and three times less likely to develop pulmonary edema. None of the "prayed for" group required intubation (being placed on a ventilator), while twelve in the other group did. Fewer in the "prayed-for" group died, although this number was not statistically significant.[5] If this had been a new wonder drug, the pharmaceutical companies would have been crawling all over themselves to patent it.

Because of the groundbreaking nature of this study, it raised as many questions as it answered. Any good study does just that. The Byrd study was not without some legitimate criticism. Because Byrd was a Christian, many felt his use of only Christian prayer groups created an intentional bias. Some believed it was an attempt to promote the idea that only "born-again" Christians had access to the holy hot line of healing. Others criticized what was called the first-name factor. Since the prayer groups were only given the first names of the patients, what would happen if there were two Johns, one in the "prayed-for" group and one in the "non-prayed-for" group? Another touted shortcoming was that outside prayer was not controlled. In other words, there was no mechanism to track whether Aunt Sally organized a prayer group at her church for Uncle Joe, completely independent of the study. And what if Uncle Joe was in the "non-prayed-for" group?

In a double-blind study published by Dr. Rogerio A. Lobo, MD, in the *Journal of Reproductive Medicine*, the success rate was seen to double when prayer was used for a group of women undergoing IVF treatment. Groups of Christians from 3 different countries prayed for 1 of the 2 groups of women undergoing IVF treatment to achieve pregnancy. The group who received prayer had a 50% pregnancy rate compared to the 26% success rate for the group who didn't receive any intercessory prayer.

In spite of the complaints and criticisms, many prominent physicians thought the study presented some valuable information. Dr. William Nolen, prominent surgeon and author, said, "It looks like this study will stand up to scrutiny. (Maybe we doctors ought to be writing on our order sheets, 'pray three times a day.' If it works. . . . It works."[6]

The largest study to date testing intercessory prayer was published in 2006 in the *American Heart Journal*. It was known as the Study of the Therapeutic Effects of Intercessory Prayer or STEP. The authors followed eighteen hundred cardiac surgery patients, dividing them into three groups: a prayed-for group who didn't know they were being prayed for, a prayed-for group who knew they were being prayed for, and a non-prayed-for group. After analyzing various factors and statistics, the authors concluded that there was no difference in any of the groups regarding outcomes and complications.

Critics of this study pointed out a variety of shortcomings in the study design and analysis, with Karl Gilberson, an editorial writer for *Science and Theology News*, stating, "I do not plan to stop praying as a result of this study, and I don't suggest anyone else stop praying either."[7] Francis MacNutt, a pioneer in the resurgence of healing and intercessory prayer, writes about this study: "Not only did the STEP study contradict our experience, it also seemed to go counter to the teachings of Jesus, 'Ask and you shall receive.'"[8] He goes on to explain this disparity by questioning the qualifications of the "pray-ers" and the design of the study. He makes a critical point in that, in his experience, intercessors must have an "expectant faith" to be effective. In other words, they must believe that when they pray real physical healing will take place. This is an important concept when contemplating the healing effect of prayer. Dr. Harold Koenig, professor of psychiatry and internal medicine at Duke University Medical Center, sums up the approach of testing prayer in humans like this: "I absolutely believe that intercessory prayer can influence medical outcomes, but I don't believe the natural methods of science can prove this."[9]

PRAYER IN NONHUMAN SYSTEMS

These criticisms illustrate the intrinsic difficulty in studying prayer in humans. There are so many factors, variables, and individual variations that it is hard (if not impossible) to eliminate these variables and only focus on the entity you are interested in: prayer, in this case.

The next logical step, given this difficulty, is to study prayer and its effects on nonhuman systems. The use of nonhuman subjects somewhat simplifies the design and increases the statistical validity. In many experiments of this nature, only the activity you are interested in testing is changed. Again, the literature on this approach is vast. It appears that there are even more published studies on prayer's healing ability on animals and plants than on people!

Dr. Dan Benor summarized the findings of many of these studies in a paper he authored. He reviewed 131 studies that specifically focused on prayer's effects on plants and animals, and in 56 he found statistically significant evidence of a positive impact on the organism.[10]

This type of study makes many people in the Christian community uncomfortable. Some feel it degrades prayer and doesn't respect the holiness of the act. I sympathize with their arguments and view these kinds of studies with skepticism. I have a theological problem with addressing prayer in nonhuman systems, and the study designs tend to skew the results based on the biases of the researcher. I put little credence on these types of studies and only present them here for completeness.

MORE QUESTIONS

After reviewing all the evidence, I was haunted by two questions: *If prayer works, why doesn't it always work?* and *Why do spiritual people get sick?* The answer to the first question lies in how I asked the question. What I was really asking was, if prayer works, why doesn't it always work *as I want it to?*

Are we so presumptuous to claim to know the mind of God? Can we begin to understand fully the purpose that God holds for us? When prayer doesn't have the expected result, do we assume God didn't hear our petitions or do we believe that we know what is best over and above a sovereign God? I suggest not. It is through faith that we understand all prayers are heard and answered. God answers prayers in ways that are not always congruent with our beliefs and demands. I am reminded of God's admonition to Job when questioned about his actions: "Will you discredit my justice and condemn me just to prove you are right? Are you as strong as God? Can you thunder with a voice like his?" (Job 40:8–9). God's character is one of love and goodness. Any answer to prayer is predicated on that foundation.

When we pray for someone to be healed, shouldn't that include not only physical healing but also healing of mind and spirit? To me, that is true healing. If we, as Christians, view death as an endpoint, if it represents a failure of healing prayer, then we are in for much disappointment. Death happens! It is a reality of the physical world we inhabit. Christians view death as the end of our physical bodies, but our soul carries on. Our struggle is not against death and disease, it is against sin and eternal separation from God.

HEALING AND DEATH

Think of the practical problems that would arise if everyone who was prayed for was miraculously healed. Not only would that selectively suspend natural law, but it would also cheapen the concept of the miraculous. Death is a natural result of physical laws, yet it is not the gauge for the success or failure of prayer. I saw a bumper sticker that read, "Eat healthy. Exercise daily. Die anyway!" That is a cynical way of viewing life, but it is steeped in truth. I'm reminded of the man who died and went to heaven. Once there, it was more magnificent than he ever imagined. He said to St. Peter, "What joy, what beauty! If I had known it was going to be this great, I would have come here years earlier."

St. Peter replied, "You would have if you hadn't eaten so many of those bran flakes!"

I am convinced that a person can physically die and yet be healed. Acceptance of this concept relies on your understanding of healing. You can be very physically ill and be healed spiritually. Dan Richardson was a devoted Christian who lost his battle with cancer at an early age. This poem was read at his funeral. The author is unknown.

> Cancer is so limited. . . .
> It cannot cripple love,
> It cannot shatter hope,
> It cannot corrode faith,
> It cannot eat away peace,
> It cannot destroy confidence,
> It cannot kill friendship,
> It cannot shut out memories,
> It cannot silence courage,
> It cannot invade the soul,
> It cannot reduce eternal life,
> It cannot quench the Spirit,
> It cannot lessen the power of the resurrection.

Cancer took his physical body, but his spirit soared.

DOES SPIRITUAL HEALTH GUARANTEE PHYSICAL HEALTH?

Why do spiritual people get sick? This is a question that many theologians have struggled with for centuries. Is illness some sort of divine punishment? The entire book of Job in the Bible addresses these questions, among others. Many illnesses are, in large part, a matter of the natural consequences of our choices. If you smoke, your risk of lung cancer skyrockets. If you don't exercise and don't eat a healthy diet, you are more likely to succumb to heart disease. These are predictable outcomes to God's unyielding natural laws. There is not a one-to-one correlation between spirituality and health. There is no question that pursuing a spiritual, prayerful life will improve one's health (mind, body, and spirit), but it does not free you from disease. Living a Christian life does not guarantee health.

Do I understand why young children get cancer? Can I make sense of the suffering of AIDS victims? Can I logically justify why bad things happen to good people? No, I can't. But I can keep from obsessing about *why* and focus on *what now*. I do not profess to know the mind of God, but I do know Paul's command in 1 Thessalonians 5:16-18: "Be cheerful no matter what; pray all the time; thank God *no matter what happens*. This is the way God wants you who belong to Christ Jesus to live" (THE MESSAGE, emphasis mine).

The story of Job gives us great practical insight into why bad things, like illness, befall good people. The book begins with the statement, "He was blameless—a man of complete integrity. He feared God and stayed away from evil" (Job 1:1). Yet tragedy after tragedy befell this spiritual man. What is the conclusion at the end of this story? It is easy to believe that we have all the answers. In reality, only God knows why things happen as they do, and we must always remember that he is in control. We are not puppets. We show our love and devotion through our decisions; however, God's love is always there, guiding events. *The Life Application Bible Commentary* puts it this way:

God is in control. In our world invaded by sin, calamity and suffering come to good and bad alike.

This does not mean that God is indifferent, uncaring, unjust, or powerless to protect us. Bad things happen because we live in a fallen world, where both believers and unbelievers are hit with the tragic consequences of sin. God allows evil for a time although he turns it around for our good (Romans 8:28). We may have no answers as to why God allows evil, but we can be sure he is all-powerful and knows what he is doing. The next time you face trials and dilemmas, see them as opportunities to turn to God for strength. You will find a God who only desires to show his love and compassion to you. If you can trust him in pain, confusion, and loneliness, you will win the victory and eliminate doubt, one of Satan's greatest footholds in your life. Make God your foundation. You can never be separated from his love.[11]

The New Testament writings and Jesus' healings also confirm that illness is not punishment from God. John 9:1–3 says: "As Jesus was walking along, he saw a man who had been blind from birth. 'Rabbi,' his disciples asked him, 'Why was this man born blind? Was it because of his own sins or his parents' sins?'

"'It was not because of his sins or his parents' sins,' Jesus answered. 'This happened so the power of God could be seen in him.'"

The story concludes as Jesus heals the blind man, fulfilling his destiny as an example of the healing power of the Christ. If I imagine myself as that blind man, I envision asking: "Why me? Why was I born blind? Why do I have to suffer this affliction?" Apparently the disciples were troubled by these same questions, and this prompted their questioning of Jesus. It is obvious from the way their query is worded that they believed, as many did then and still do today, that the only understandable explanation for this man's infirmity lay in some defect in his or his parents' character. In other words, his blindness was a punishment for some unknown sin. Jesus quickly countered this belief by eloquently explaining that the blindness had nothing to do with sins or behavior. He stated that God knew the true meaning of this illness, and it was to illuminate the glory of God through the healing.

Dr. Larry Dossey states, "Sickly saints and healthy sinners show us that there is no invariable, one-to-one relationship between one's level of spiritual attainment and the degree of one's physical health. It is obvious that one can achieve great spiritual heights and still get very sick."[12]

Remember, healing is much more than just ridding the body of disease; it is balancing mind, body, and spirit.

FRUITS OF PRAYER

The Coping with Cancer study, a multi-institutional investigation of advanced cancer patients and their main care-givers recently concluded that of 230 patients surveyed, the vast major-ity—88%—considered religion to be at least somewhat important. But nearly half said their spiritual needs were largely or entirely unmet by a religious community, and 72% felt those needs were similarly unaddressed by the medical system. The findings also indi-cated that greater spiritual support from religious organizations and medical service providers was strongly linked to better quality of life for patients, even after other factors were taken into account.[13]

What benefits do we see in prayer? If we don't know or can't predict results, then why pray? In simple terms, it's not about getting. It is about learning to achieve a state of prayerfulness—a state where you be-come open to God's love and healing presence. Jane Vennard, in an audio-tape called "Intercessory Prayer," talks about the "fruits" of prayer.[14] I love the analogy of fruit because it is a substance that must be cultivated and nourished to grow, and in turn can serve as nourishment to others. Fully developed, it can even seed the growth of additional fruit. Prayer is much like this. She states that one of the fruits of prayer is a God-centered existence. God is responsible for all we are, have, and will be, and through prayer we remind ourselves of our dependence on him. Praying for healing will refocus us on the Healer instead of the disease. It puts God in the center of our lives and encourages us to replace our egocentric thoughts with those of divine grace. It paves the way for healing.

The second fruit of healing prayer is compassion. Through prayer we embrace a heightened level of compassion for those about whom we pray. This takes the form of empathy, truly feeling the needs of the afflicted. Healing prayer brings hope. When suicide survivors are interviewed, inevitably they report reaching a state of hopelessness that drove them to the attempt on their life. There is no greater feeling of desperation than being without hope. Praying for yourself or others restores hope, perpetuates hope, and, in some cases, creates hope.

Ms. Vennard states that another fruit of intercessory prayer is action. Whether it is serving meals to the homeless or helping a tornado victim find parts of a ravaged home, prayer can spur us to action. The action itself may be a form of prayer. We may join a protest for basic human rights or volunteer at a hospice. Prayer gives us direction, provides focus, and forces us to listen. In the silence of prayer, the call to action can be deafening.

Finally, prayer emphasizes thankfulness, the attitude of gratitude. Giving thanks to God for healing reminds us where the healing originates. It is a simple concept, but one I find helpful in centering my faith. It is a statement of faith. I believe; therefore, I thank and praise. Only a fool would thank someone for something they knew they wouldn't receive.

HOW TO

Richard Foster, in his book *Prayer*, writes, "God, I have a thousand arguments against healing prayer. You are the one argument for it. . . . you win!"[15] He then explains his approach to praying for healing. He says this is not a how-to guide for healing prayer but a template to build on. His ideas are useful as a guide to aid in all communication with God, not just specific to healing. He describes four steps to healing prayer: listening, asking, knowing, and thanking.

Listening is vital to effective communication with God or anyone else. One of the monumental apprehensions people have about prayer is "doing it right." They are afraid that they will not say the right thing or even know what to say. You cannot pray wrong! Just the act of praying makes it right. You don't have to say anything! Just be quiet and listen. This may be more difficult for some than speaking.

Being quiet does not come naturally for many people, but listening can be a learned behavior. Listen to people and they will tell you their prayer needs. First-year medical students are told that simply listening to patients will provide the diagnosis of their problem the vast majority of times. Practice being still in prayer. It will take the pressure off, and you may be surprised at what you hear. In his book mentioned above,

Richard Foster talks about his own intercessory prayer experience. He says, "After prayer for my immediate family, I wait quietly until individuals or situations spontaneously rise to my awareness. I then offer these to God, listening to see if any special discernment comes to guide the content of the prayer."[16]

Ask God for healing for yourself and others. God knows your needs, so this is not attempting to relay new information. Rather, asking is both an act of faith and a reminder of the needs of others. By asking, you crystallize your thoughts and focus on what is important. When we become clear on the needs, asking invites healing to emerge. It opens our hearts and minds to the healing love that is always right there. It is okay to ask.

Father Arthur Tonne relates the story of a mother who told her young son to go to bed and be sure to say his prayers and ask God to make him a good boy. The boy's father, passing by the bedroom, overheard his son praying: "And God, make me a good boy if you can; and if you can't, don't worry about it, 'cause I'm having fun the way I am."

God wants us to ask. Jesus said, "Keep on asking, and you will receive what you ask for. Keep on seeking, and you will find. Keep on knocking, and the door will be opened to you. For everyone who asks, receives. Everyone who seeks, finds. And to everyone who knocks, the door will be opened" (Matthew 7:7–8).

A well-known motivational speaker's favorite phrase is "Know your outcome." Here, "know" is much more than a belief. It is that feeling that starts in the bottom of your toes and slowly fills every molecule of your being. We know with our whole person: body, mind, and spirit. This is a step of assurance. In this sense it is almost analogous to faith. "Faith is the confidence [knowing] that what we hope for will actually happen; it gives us assurance about things we cannot see" (Hebrews 11:1).

The final step is thanks, the attitude of gratitude. Giving thanks for what we know is to be. Praise and prayer are like peanut butter and jelly; they just go together! Gratitude humbles us and reminds us whose we are.

PRAYER WORKS

Emily and Stan, a young couple, were expecting their second child. Their firstborn was five-year-old Sammy. During the present pregnancy, Sammy would crawl up next to his mother and rub her ever-expanding tummy and sing to his future sibling. It was his way of getting to know the unborn baby. This continued throughout the uneventful pregnancy until labor ensued. The labor was short, yet at the end Emily developed some problems that necessitated an emergency C-section.

The joy and anticipation of the new arrival was somewhat dampened by the news that the new baby girl showed signs of an infection. The little girl, whom they named Sally, was taken to the neonatal intensive care nursery in this small hospital to be watched more closely. After a few hours the pediatrician came to Emily's room and told her that the little baby had taken a turn for the worse. They were going to have to transfer the baby to a specialized nursery downtown for more intensive care. You can only imagine the devastation and apprehension both Emily and Stan felt as they watched their newborn being wheeled into the ambulance for the transfer.

After a day at the new hospital, the neonatologist spoke to Emily as she was visiting Sally. "We are very concerned about Sally," he said slowly. "The next twenty-four hours are critical. She could turn around, or she could get a lot worse. I just thought you should know to be able to tell any family members to stay close by."

Emily could read between the lines. She knew that the doctor was telling her that her child might not make it. Then it occurred to her that Sammy had not yet seen his baby sister. She decided that if there was a chance baby Sally was going to die, she had to get Sammy in to see her.

The neonatal intensive care unit is a very mechanical, sterile environment, and small children are not allowed to visit because of the risk of infection. This didn't dissuade Emily as she dressed Sammy in a little rolled-up scrub suit and put on a mask and walked into the unit. The nurses went berserk! But when they realized what was going on, they reluctantly agreed to the brief visit. Babies in the NICU lie in beds that are up on pedestals to allow the nurses to work with them more easily.

They retrieved a couple of boxes for Sammy to stand on, and he climbed up and peered over the bassinet for a first look at his new sister.

To most, the sight of a little baby with a tube in her throat and IV lines from her arms would be frightening. Not to Sammy. He peered intently at Sally and then spontaneously reached down and grabbed her tiny hand and began to sing, just as he had done to his mommy's tummy. "You are my sunshine, my only sunshine. You make me happy when skies are gray. You'll never know, dear, how much I love you. Please, God, don't take my sister away."

The nurses were the first to notice a difference in the baby. That evening Sally's vital signs stabilized and her temperature became normal. She was able to breathe on her own within twenty-four hours and was discharged home two days later, a healthy, happy baby sister. The local newspaper that had followed the story called it a miracle; the doctors and nurses all called it a miracle. I call it the healing power of prayer.

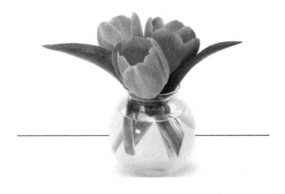

CELEBRATE!

Where do you want to be in five years? What is your mission? What is your purpose and vision? Do you want to live as you are now, or do you want something different?

Proverbs 29:18 says that "where there is no vision, the people perish" (KJV). A vision is knowledge of who you are and what you want to be and accomplish. To know your outcome is to see the path to your vision. Imagine how difficult it would be to plan a weeklong trip or vacation and not know your destination. You wouldn't know how long to allot for travel. You wouldn't know where to make nighttime hotel reservations. You wouldn't even know which way to turn out of the driveway.

So it is with life. If you don't have a clear picture of where you want to go, you will be relegated to wandering aimlessly, searching for an unclear, unidentified destination. If you don't have an acute understanding of what you want your life to be, then you tend to experience the frustration of directionless decisions.

Do you know how you want to spend the third of your life during menopause and beyond? Have you envisioned how this time, whether you are in your forties dealing with PMS or later in perimenopause, can be a celebration rather than a struggle to survive?

I challenge you to begin today to create the vision of a fulfilling and purposeful life. This first step is essential, for it creates the atmosphere in which all your thoughts and actions will be nurtured. Saturate this vision with prayer. Let prayer be the canvas on which you paint your midlife. No matter the form, color, or style of the picture, the canvas is always there, underlying every stroke, supporting every dream.

Mission and purpose can come in prayer. It can come through action, reading, meditation, and discussion. How you formulate your mission is unique, yet the common denominator is prayer. Missions are not complicated. Jesus said, "I came that they may have life, and have it abundantly" (John 10:10 NASB). Nehemiah's goal was simply to rebuild the wall of Jerusalem. The twelve apostles shared a common mission to go out and teach what they had learned. Mother Teresa's purpose was to show love and compassion to the poorest of the poor. Your mission can be just as simple and no less grand.

This book is a springboard. My heartfelt prayer is that you will find some kernel of wisdom to stimulate you to think and act. But don't stop there. This is only a door that opens to a vast storehouse of discoveries awaiting you on your journey.

Dr. Wayne Sotile, speaker and author, talks about stress in his book *Supercouple Syndrome*. He feels many of us live in times of high stress and low control. This is a toxic stress that can overwhelm our physical and spiritual well-being. This certainly describes menopause for many women, a time of many stresses and loss of control. In fact, times of toxic stress are associated with the highest rate of divorce, illness, and depression for women.

Consider the idea of high stress/low control with respect to menopause. What I find interesting (and what I hope you understand after reading this book) is that both of these situations—high stress and low control—are situations that are dictated by your thoughts. You have already seen how stress is based on your perceptions. What is stressful to one may not be stressful to another; the difference is how each person perceives the stressor. The loss of control during menopause is often secondary to the ignorance of choices and a lack of understanding of physiology. The preceding chapters have illustrated how to take back control of your life. You have guidelines to reshape your perception of stress, and you can alter the reality of your situation. It begins with knowing your destination. That often is determined by answering the "W" questions at the beginning of this chapter. If you can determine where you want to go, then the "how to get there" will follow.

We've discussed one path to a celebration of midlife: attitude, aptitude, action, and apothecary. Begin with the intention of knowing your outcome. Know that God has a plan for you, and he will see you through. Be open to his guidance. Immerse yourself in prayer and meditation to determine your path. Listen. Hear God. Cultivate a personal relationship with him. Educate yourself. Use every resource available to know options and to make decisions. Bathe yourself in knowledge and wisdom from Scripture, friends, family, doctors, books, seminars, CDs, and experience. Make it an adventure! Take action. Use the knowledge that you acquire. Embrace exercise, vitamins, herbs, and nutrition, and eliminate those behaviors you know to be harmful.

Enjoy life and all that is here for you as you maximize your gifts. That implies action and commitment. This book is a call to action. Immobility, inaction, stagnation, and paralysis are your enemies.

Every action begins with a thought. Every great deed is predicated on a conviction. The only true failure in life is not taking action, not trying anything new, or fearing success. When you do something to improve your feelings or thoughts, there are only two possible outcomes: either you accomplish your task or you don't. And if you don't, you haven't failed. You have just learned another way not to get the results you want!

Everyone is unique. There are no two women who will waltz through midlife with the same dance steps. Each dance is special and your own. It stands to reason that not all women will benefit from every technique or recommendation in this book. This variation does not invalidate the suggestions. Take what feels right to you, try it, and evaluate whether it is accomplishing your goal. Is it eliminating the hot flashes? Is it improving libido? If not, try something else. Don't relinquish all other options. God will not abandon you, no matter what road you take.

To create a space for joy in menopause, do the following:

Make a plan; set a goal. Decide where you want your life to go. Suffuse the process with prayer. There is nothing fiendish in visualizing the kind of life you want. Trust in God to open your heart and mind to the possibilities. He came in the person of Jesus so that you may have life and have it *abundantly*. Listen, believe, meditate, visualize, and pray.

Don't lose sight of your mission. It is so easy to get caught up in the hurry sickness of our times. Pay the bills. Drive the carpool. Climb the ladder. Volunteer here. Hurry over there. Every decision of importance you make should be measured by the standard of your vision. Does this action bring me closer to God? Does this activity support my calling?

Remember that taking action drives the engine of happiness. I suppose some could be content spending hours doing nothing. As I said earlier, a little loafing every now and then is refreshing, but it is not an effective lifestyle. The evidence is overwhelming that if you want to live a long and happy life, you must stay active, both mentally and physically. The realities of aging place some limits, yet the greatest limiting factor is that which we place on ourselves.

Constantly evaluate what you are doing. Is this herb working? Is my prayer life what I want it to be? Am I losing the weight I want to? Do I sleep better at night? Never stop asking questions. Always reassess every major decision to see if it (a) accomplishes the intended goal, and (b) is consistent with your beliefs and integrity. If your actions are not getting you where you want to be, change course. Do something different; try a new angle. There are no failures, just different ways of doing things.

Listen with a discerning ear to others. A fool hears only what she wants to and nothing she should. When the student is ready, the teacher will appear. Understand that most information you receive from the media has an agenda. It may be a positive, spiritually driven agenda, but a bias always exists. Be open, but be critical.

Partner with someone; be it your spouse, a good friend, a support group, or your doctor. Share your mission and your vision for this transition and beyond. They will keep you accountable and will be supportive during the inevitable trials and tribulations.

Have fun! Don't ever underestimate the healing potential of good times. Laughter truly can be wonderful medicine. Norman Cousins knew it, Patch Adams knew it, and Solomon knew it. Now you know it, so laugh three times a day. Doctor's orders!

Respect the healing triad: mind, body, and spirit. Health means wholeness, and wholeness is a balance of all three. Remember the baby's mobile, where none is isolated and each one exerts its influence on the others.

Never stop learning. I am continually amazed at how much I don't know! It used to bother me, but now I see it as a glorious opportunity to discover. Never stop saying "Aha!" Recapture the wonder of childhood where every day is an adventure.

Always maintain the attitude of gratitude. Thank God at every opportunity for blessing you with life and the ability to make it a wondrous journey. All we are and can be comes from God, and he even gave us an example to follow. Even in the darkest hours, even in the lowest points, even in the hottest flashes, he is there saying, "Come on, Sally. Come on, Julie. Come on, Barbara. Walk with me."

NOTES

INTRODUCTION

1. Tom Minnery, *Why You Can't Stay Silent* (Carol Stream, IL: Tyndale House, 2002).
2. B. Ettinger, D.K. Li, and R. Klien, "Continuation of postmenopausal hormone replacement therapy in cyclic and continuous regimens," *Menopause* 3 (1996): 185–89.
3. "Menopause," *Pharmasave.com, http://content.nhiondemand.com/psv/HC2.asp?objID=1002 36&cType=hc,* (accessed August 31, 2007).
4. S.I. McMillen, *None of These Diseases* (Grand Rapids, MI: Baker Book House, 1963), 15.
5. *Journal of the General Conference of the United Methodist Church,* April 1972, Atlanta, GA.
6. Michael D. Lemonick, "Score One for the Bible," *Time,* March 5, 1990.
7. P. Barnes, E. Powell-Griner, K. McFann, R. Nahin, "Complementary and Alternative Medicine Use Among Adults: United States, 2002," *CDC Advance Data Report #343,* May 27, 2004.

THE HEALING TRIAD

1. Gail Sheehy, *The Silent Passage,* rev. ed. (New York: Random House, 1998), author notes.
2. North American Menopause Society, *Menopause* pamphlet, 2005.
3. Farah Kostreski, "A Major Trend," *Ob-Gyn News,* December 15, 1998, 6.
4. "The Beginning of the End?" November 2003, *www.premarin.org.*
5. Sara Selis, "Drug Promotion Expenditure Quantified," *Stanford Medicine Magazine,* Fall 2003, *http://stanford.edu/2003fall/scope-fall2003.html.*

COMPLEMENTARY MEDICINE AND THE BIBLE

1. "Herbal Medical: An Overview" University of Maryland Medical Center webpage *www.unm.edu.*

2. W. Sampson, et al., "Acupuncture: The Position Paper of the National Council Against Health Fraud," *Clinical Journal of Pain* 7 (1991): 162-166.
3. Virginia Owens, *Daughters of Eve* (Colorado Springs: Navpress Publishing Group, 1995), 26.
4. Henry Curwin, ed., *A Johnson Sampler* (Boston: David R. Godine Publishers, 2002), 24.
5. Stanley Turkel, "The U.S. Population Age 65 and Over Is Expected to Double in the Next 25 Years," July 18, 2006, *www.hospitalitynet.org/news/4028342.html*.
6. Margaret Lock, "Encounters With Aging: Mythologies of Menopause in Japan and North America," *Pacific Affairs* 68, no. 1 (Spring, 1995), 123-124.
7. E. Brooks Holifield, *Health and Medicine in the Methodist Tradition* (New York: Crossroad Publishers, 1986), 6.
8. Mitch Albom, *Tuesdays with Morrie* (New York: Doubleday, 1997), 43.
9. Ibid., 57.

THE PERPLEXING PERIMENOPAUSE

1. Jimmy Carter, *An Hour Before Daylight: Memories of a Rural Boyhood* (New York: Simon and Schuster, 2001), vi.
2. North American Menopause Society Newsletter, June 1999.
3. H. Norman Wright, *Simplify Your Life* (Wheaton, IL: Tyndale House, 1997), 6.
4. Zig Ziglar, *Over the Top* (Nashville: Thomas Nelson, 1997).
5. Randall S. Hansen, PhD, "Is Your Life in Balance?" *Quintessential Careers, www.quintcareers.com/work-life_balance_quiz.html*.
6. "Women's Health Initiative" study from National Institute of Health, *www.nhlbc.nilt.gov/whi*.
7. Neil Warren, *Finding Contentment* (Nashville: Thomas Nelson Publishers, 1997).

MENOPAUSE: PUBERTY WITH EXPERIENCE

1. Max Lucado, *He Still Moves Stones* (Dallas: Word Publishing, 1993).
2. "Book of Ruth," *Wikipedia,* September 2007, *http://en.wikipedia.org/wiki/Book_of_Ruth*.
3. *NIV Life Application Bible* (Wheaton, IL: Tyndale House, 1988), 423.
4. Robert L. Hubbard Jr., *The Book of Ruth* (Grand Rapids, MI: William B. Eerdmans Publishing Company, 1988), 14.

THE FOUR A's

1. Laurie Gottlieb, *Dreams Have No Expiration Date, n.p., n.d.*
2. "Christian Motivation for Daily Living," Ziglar training systems (Dallas, TX, 1998).
3. Charles Swindoll, quoted from *Christian Reader* 33, no. 4.
4. Positive Psychology Center, University of Pennsylvania, *www.ppc.sas.upenn.edu/*
5. Bob Phillips, *Phillips' Book of Great Thoughts and Funny Sayings* (Wheaton, IL: Tyndale House, 1993), 28.
6. Rob Stein, "Researchers Look at Prayer and Healing," *Washington Post,* Friday, March 24, 2006, A01.
7. "Placebo," *Wikipedia*, September 11, 2007, *http://en.wikipedia.org/wiki/Placebo_(origins_of_technical_term)*.
8. Dr. Andrew Grimes, Fifty-fourth American Society for Reproductive Medicine meeting, San Francisco, CA, July 1998.

TREATMENT OPTIONS: HORMONES

1. Barbara Seaman, *The Greatest Experiment Ever Performed on Women: Exploding the Estrogen Myth* (New York: Hyperion, 2003), 7.

2. National Women's Health Network, "The Truth About Hormone Replacement Therapy: How to Break Free From the Medical Myths of Menopause," 2002, 160-161.

3. Kaiser Permanente Health System Statistics, "A Survey of Hormone Therapy Use," 1999.

4. "The Fortune 500: Honey, I Shrunk the Profits," *Fortune,* 147, no. 7 (April 17, 2003), F-59.

5. Jacques Rossouw, MD, "The Heart and Estrogen/Progestin Replacement Study," *Journal of American Medical Association* (August 19, 1998).

6. Committee Opinion #322, "Compounded Bioidentical Hormones," *Obstetrics & Gynecology*, November 2005, 2.

7. *1999 Physician's Desk Reference.*

8. "Nature's Healing Pharmacy," Green Medicine, *www.nps.gov/plants/medicinal/plants.htm.*

9. Center for Disease Control, MMWR weekly newsletter, March 10, 1989.

10. Collaborative Group on Hormonal Factors in Breast Cancer, *The Lancet* 350 (1997): 1047.

11. B.K. Armstrong, "Oestrogen therapy after menopause," *Medical Journal of Australia* 148, no. 5 (1988): 213–14.

12. W.D. Dupont and D.L. Page, "Menopausal estrogen replacement therapy and breast cancer," *Archives of Internal Medicine* 151 (1991): 67–72.

13. K.K. Steinberg, S.B. Thacker, S.J. Smith, et al., "A meta-analysis of the effect of estrogen replacement therapy on the risk of breast cancer," *Journal of American Medical Association* 265 (1991): 1985–90.

14. Graham Colditz, "Hormone replacement therapy and the risk of breast cancer: results from epidemiological studies," *American Journal of Obstetrics and Gynecology* 168 (1993): 1473–80.

15. J.L. Stanford et al., "Combined estrogen and progesterone replacement therapy in relation to risk of breast cancer in middle age women," *Journal of American Medical Association* 274 (1989): 137–42: D.W Kaufman, "Estrogen replacement therapy and the risk of breast cancer: results from the case controlled surveillance study," *American Journal of Epidemiology* 134 (1991): 1375–85; and J.R. Palmer, et al., "Breast cancer risk after estrogen replacement therapy: results from the Toronto breast cancer study," *American Journal of Epidemiology* 134 (1991): 1386–95.

16. "Women's Health Initiative Findings," University of Washington School of Medicine Department of Obstetrics and Gynecology newsletter, August 15, 2003.

17. "About Breast Cancer," Breastcancer.org, 2006, *www.breastcancer.org/about_us/press_kit/cancer_facts.jsp.*

18. Colditz, 1473–80.

19. The writing group of the PEPI trial, "Effect of estrogen on heart disease risk factors in postmenopausal women: The postmenopausal estrogen/progesterone interventions trial," *Journal of American Medical Association* 273 (1995): 199–208.

TREATMENT OPTIONS: COMPLEMENTARY APPROACHES

1. Lotke and Albertazzi, "The effect of dietary soy supplementation on hot flushes," *Obstetrics and Gynecology* (1998): 6–11.
2. Ibid.
3. Messina, "The role of soy products in reducing cancer," *Journal of the National Cancer Institute* 83 (1991): 541–46.
4. J.W. Anderson, "Meta-analysis on the effects of soy protein intake on serum lipids," *New England Journal of Medicine* 353 (1995): 276–82.
5. Aldercreutz, "Phytoestrogens in western diseases," *Annals of Medicine* 29 (1997): 95–120.
6. Adapted from K. Reinli and G. Block, "Phytoestrogen content of foods—a compendium of literature values," *Nutrition and Cancer* 26 (1996): 123-48.
7. R.S. Finkler, "The effect of vitamin E in menopause," *Journal of Clinical Endocrinol Metabolism* 9 (1949): 89–94.
8. S. Lieberman, "A review of the effectiveness of Cimicifuga Racemosa for the symptoms of menopause," *Journal of Women's Health* 5 (1998): 529.
9. E. Lehmann-Willenbrock and H. H. Riedel, "Clinical and endocrinological examinations concerning therapy of climacteric symptoms following hysterectomy with remaining ovaries," *American Journal of Health-System Pharmacy* 110 (1998): 611–18.
10. Warneche, "Influencing menopausal symptoms with a phytotherapautic agent," *Med Welt* 36 (1985): 871-74.
11. N. Beuscher, "Cimicifuga Racemosa," *Phytotherapie* 16 (1995): 301–10.
12. Report on the Tenth World Congress on Fertility and Sterility, June 2002. Berlin, Germany.
13. Bob Murray, PhD, and Alicia Fortinberry, MS, "Depression Facts and Stats," Uplift Program, January 15, 2005, *www.upliftprogram.com/depression_stats.html#1*.
14. Stoll, "Phytopharmacuetical influences on atrophic vaginal epithelium," *Therapeuticum* 1 (1987): 23-31.
15. Covert Bailey, *Smart Exercise* (New York: Houghton Mifflin, 1994), 271.
16. James A. Blumenthal, PhD, Michael A. Babyak, PhD, Kathleen A. Moore, PhD, et al., "Effects of Exercise Training on Older Patients With Major Depression," *Archives of Internal Medicine* 159, no. 19 (October 25, 1999): 2349–56.
17. W. Poldinger, Calanchini, and W. Scwartz, "A functional dimensional approach to depression: serotonin deficiency as a target syndrome in a comparison of 5-HTP and fluvoxamine," *Psychopathology* 24 (1991): 53–81.
18. Murray, *Encyclopedia of Natural Medicine*, 397.
19. E.V. Vorbach, W. D. Hubner, and K. H. Arnoldt, "Effectiveness and tolerance of the Hypericumextract LI 160 in comparison with Imipramine: randomized double-blind study with 135 outpatients," *Journal of Geriatric Psychiatry Neurology* 17 (1994): 519–23.
20. K. Linde, G. Ramirez, and C.D. Mulrow, "Saint-John's-wort for depression: an overview and meta-analysis of randomized clinical trials," *British Medical Journal* 313 (1996): 253–58.
21. I. Hindmarch and Z. Subhan, "The psychopharmalogical effects of Ginkgo Biloba extract in normal healthy volunteers," *International Journal of Clinical Pharmacology* 4 (1984): 89–93.
22. P.L. Lebars, et al., "A placebo controlled double-blind randomized trial of an extract of Gingko Biloba for dementia," *Journal of American Medical Association* 278 (1997): 1327–32.

23. National Health Interview Survey, 2005.

24. M.S. Santos, F. Ferreira, and A.P. Cunha, "A liquid extract of valerian influences the transport of GABA in synaptosomes," *Planta Medica* 60 (1994): 278–79.

25. G. Warnecke, "Neurovegetative dystonia in the female climacteric: studies on the clinical efficacy and the tolerance of Kava extract," *Fortschr Med* 109 (1991): 120-22.

26. J.K. Walsh and C.L. Engelhardt, "The direct economic costs of insomnia in the United States for 1995," *Sleep* 22, no. 2 (May 1, 1999): 386-93.

27. A. Soulairac and H. Lambinet, "Clinical studies of the effect of the serotonin precursor L-5 Hydroxytryptophan on sleep disorders," *Schweizerische Rundschau für Medizin Praxis* 77 (1988): 19–23.

28. P. Leatherwood et al., "Aqueous extract of valerian root improves sleep quality in man," *Pharmacology Biochemistry and Behavior* 17 (1982): 65–71.

29. O. Lindahl and L. Lindwall, "Double-blind study of a valerian preparation," *Pharmacology Biochemistry and Behavior* 32 (1989): 1065–6.

30. R. Nave, R. Peled, and P. Lavie, "Melatonin in improving evening napping," *European Journal of Pharmacology* 275 (1995): 213–16.

31. National Association of Continence, December 4, 2006, *www.nafc.org/statistics/index.htm.*

32. I. Ofek, et al., "Anti-escherichia activity of cranberry and blueberry juices," *New England Journal of Medicine* 324 (1991): 1599.

33. B. Larrson, A. Jonasson, and S. Fianu, "Prophylactic effect of Uva-E on women with recurrent cystitis: a preliminary report," *Current Therapeutic Research* 53 (1993): 441–43.

34. H. H. Amin, T. V. Subbaiah, and K. M. Abbasi, "Berberine sulfate antimicrobial activity, bioassay, and mode of action," *Canadian Journal of Microbiology* 15 (1969): 1067–76.

35. N. Bellamy, W. C. Buchanon, and E. Grace, "A double-blind randomized controlled study of isoxican versus piroxicam in elderly patients with osteoarthritis of the hip and knee," *British Journal of Clinical Pharmacology* 22 (1986): 1495.

EXERCISE: SWEATING WITH THE OLDIES

1. "The Muscular System," Drstandley.com, *www.drstandley.com/bodysystems_muscular.shtml.*

2. Covert Bailey, *Smart Exercise*, (New York: Houghton Mifflin, 1994), 26.

3. J. Ron Eaker, *Fat-Proof Your Family* (Minneapolis: Bethany House, 2007), 19.

4. Bailey, 17.

5. The Ramblers, *www.ramblers.org.uk.*

6. George Sheehan, *Running and Being* (New York: Simon and Schuster, 1978), 4.

7. Alice Feinstein, ed., *Training the Body to Cure Itself* (Emmaus, PA: Rodale Press, 1992), 3.

8. National Institute on Aging Guide for Exercise, NIA publication, December, 2005.

9. Baylor College of Medicine Office of Health Promotion, *Vitality, Vim, and Vigor: Six steps to more energy* (Baylor Plaza, Houston: Baylor College of Medicine Office of Health Promotion).

10. Feinstein, 19.

11. "Varicose Veins and Spider Veins," U.S. Department of Health and Human Services, *www.4woman.gov/faq/varicose.htm.*

12. Feinstein, 221.

13. Ibid., 222.

DIET AND NUTRITION: EAT SMART—LIVE LONG

1. Center for Disease Control Web site, *www.cdc.gov/nccdphp/dnpa/obesity*, May 2006.
2. The Nutrition Screening Initiative, 1010 Wisconsin Avenue, NW, Suite 800, Washington, DC 20007.
3. *NIV Life Application Bible* (Wheaton, Ill.: Tyndale House, 1988), 2070.

LOST LIBIDO: WHAT TO DO WHEN YOUR SEX DRIVE HAS DRIVEN OFF

1. P.M. Sarrel, "Sexuality in the middle years," *Obstetrics and Gynecology Clinics of North America* 14 (1987): 49–62.
2. Roe Gallo and Stephen Zocchi, *Overcoming the Myths of Aging* (San Francisco: Roe Gallo Publishing).
3. Sarrel, 60.
4. Stolze, "An alternative to treat menopausal complaints," *Obstetrics and Gynecology* 3 (1982): 674.
5. K.A. Hanson and S. Tho, "Androgen and bone health," *Seminars in Reproductive Endocrinology* 16 (1998): 129–30.
6. R.D. Dickerman, W.J. McConathy, and N.Y. Zacharrah, "Testosterone, sex hormone binding globulin, lipoproteins and vascular disease risk," *Journal of Cardiovascular Risk* 4 (1997): 363–66.

OSTEOPOROSIS: SKELETON SKILLS

1. The 2004 Surgeon General's report on Bone Health and Osteoporosis, 1–4.
2. National Osteoporosis Foundation, *www.nof.org/osteoporosis/diseasefacts.htm*.
3. G.P. Dalsky, K.S. Stocke, A.A. Ehsani, E. Slatopolsky, W.C. Lee, and S.J. Birge, "Weight-bearing exercise training and lumbar bone mineral content in postmenopausal women," *Annals of Internal Medicine* 108 (1988): 824-8.
4. A. Marsh, et al., "Bone mineral mass in lactovegetarians and omniverous adults," *American Journal of Clinical Nutrition* 37 (1983): 453–56.
5. L. Cohen and R. Kitzes, "Infrared spectroscopy and magnesium content of bone mineral in osteoporotic women," *Israel Journal of Medical Sciences* 17 (1981): 1123–25.
6. G.E. Abraham and H. Grewal, "A total dietary program emphasizing magnesium instead of calcium," *Journal of Reproductive Medicine* 35 (1990): 503–7.
7. W.S. McKane, et al., "Role of calcium intake in modulating age-related increases in parathyroid function and bone resorption," *Journal of Clinical Endocrinol Metabolism* 81 (1996): 1699–703.
8. NIH consensus conference, "Osteoporosis," *Journal of American Medical Association* 252 (1984): 799–802.
9. Katherine Zeratsky, "Calcium Supplements: Which type of calcium is best?" MayoClinic.com, *www.mayoclinic.com/health/calcium-supplements/AN00964*.
10. M.S. Christensen, C. Hagan, and C. Christensen, "Dose response evaluation of cyclic estrogen\gestigen in postmenopausal women placebo controlled trial of its gynecologic and metabolic actions," *American Journal of Obstetrics and Gynecology* 144 (1982): 873–79.

THE HEALING POWER OF PRAYER

1. Harold G. Koenig, Michael E. McCullough, David B. Larson, *The Handbook of Religion and Health* (Oxford University Press, 2000), 24.

2. B. Garia Pena, G. Taylor, D. Lund, "Appendicitis Revisited: New Insights into an Age-Old Problem," *Contemporary Pediatrics*, September 1999, 1168.

3. "Is Prayer in Workplace Allowed by Law?" All About Popular Issues, *www.allaboutpopularissues.org/prayer-in-the-workplace-faq.htm.*

4. Larry Dossey, *Prayer Is Good Medicine* (New York: HarperSanFrancisco, 1996), 10.

5. R. Byrd, "Positive therapeutic effects of intercessory prayer in a coronary care unit population," *Southern Medical Journal* 81, no. 7 (1989): 826–29.

6. Dale Matthews, *The Faith Factor* (New York: Viking, 1999), 199.

7. K.Giberson, "The Great Value of Nothing," *Science and Theology News*, May 2006, 4.

8. F. MacNutt, "Does It Make Any Difference Who Prays for My Healing?" *The Healing Line* newsletter, June 2005.

9. C. Casatelli, "Study Casts Doubt on Medicinal Use of Prayer," *Science and Theology News*, May 2006, 5.

10. D.J. Benor, "Survey of spiritual healing research," *Complementary Medicine Research* 4, no. 3 (1990), 9–33.

11. *NIV Life Application Bible* (Wheaton, IL: Tyndale House, 1988), 896.

12. Larry Dossey, *Healing Words* (New York: HarperSanFrancisco, 1993), 15.

13. Tracy A. Balboni, Lauren C. Vanderwerker, Susan D. Block, M. Elizabeth Paulk, Christopher S. Lathan, et al., "Religiousness and Spiritual Support Among Advanced Cancer Patients and Associations With End-of-Life Treatment Preferences and Quality of Life," *Journal of Clinical Oncology* 25, no. 5 (February 10, 2007): 555-560.

14. Jane Vennard, "Intercessory Prayer," Sounds True Audio, Boulder, CO, 1996.

15. R. Foster, *Prayer* (New York: HarperSanFrancisco, 1992), 216.

16. Ibid., 200.

ADDITIONAL READING

Herbs and Nutraceuticals

Colbin, Annemarie. *Food and Healing*. New York: Ballantine Books, 1986.

Dorian, Terry. *Health Begins in Him*. Lafayette, LA: Huntington House, 1995.

Fugh-Berman, Adriane. *Alternative Medicine*. Baltimore, MD: Williams and Wilkins, 1996.

Gazella, Karolyn A. *Professional's Guide to Natural Healing*. Green Bay, WI: Impakt Communications, 1997.

Gladster, Rosemary. *Herbal Healing for Women*. New York: Simon and Schuster, 1993.

Jensen, Bernard. *Foods That Heal*. Garden City, NY: Avery Publishing Group, 1993.

Murray, Michael, and Joseph Pizzorno. *Encyclopedia of Natural Medicine*. Rocklin, CA: Prima Health, 1998.

PDR for Herbal Medicines. Montvale, NJ: Medical Economics Company, 1998.

Vogel, H.C.A. *The Nature Doctor*. New Canaan, CN: Keats Publishing, 1991.

Prayer

Breathnach, Sarah. *Simple Abundance*. New York: Warner Books, 1995.

Dossey, Larry. *Healing Words*. New York: HarperSanFrancisco, 1993.

Dossey, Larry. *Prayer Is Good Medicine*. New York: HarperSanFrancisco, 1996.

Foster, Richard. *Prayer: Finding the Heart's True Home*. New York: Harper SanFrancisco, 1992.

God's Little Devotional Book II. Tulsa, OK: Honor Books, 1997.

Koenig, Harold G. *The Healing Power of Faith*. New York: Simon and Schuster, 1999.

Owings, Timothy. *Hearing God in a Noisy World*. Macon, GA: Smyth and Helwys Publishing, 1998.

Hormones

Laux, Marcus, and Christine Conrad. *Natural Woman, Natural Menopause*. New York: HarperCollins, 1997.

Nachtigall, Lila, and Joan Rattner Heilman. *Estrogen: The Facts Can Change Your Life*. New York: HarperPerennial, 1995.

Humor

Adams, Patch. *House Calls*. San Francisco: Robert Reed Publishers, 1998.

Johnson, Barbara. *Living Somewhere Between Estrogen and Death*. Dallas: Word Publishing, 1997.

Klein, Allen. *The Healing Power of Humor*. Los Angeles: Jeremy Tarcher, Inc., 1989.

Samra, Cal, and Rose Samra. *More Holy Humor*. Nashville: Thomas Nelson Publishers, 1997.

Exercise

Bailey, Covert. *The New Fit or Fat*. New York: Houghton Mifflin, 1991.

Bailey, Covert. *Smart Exercise*. New York: Houghton Mifflin, 1994.

Nutrition

Eaker, J. Ron *Fat-Proof Your Family*. Minneapolis: Bethany House Publishers, 2007.

McMillen, S.I. *None of These Diseases*. Grand Rapids, MI: Baker Books, 1984.

Russell, Rex. *What the Bible Says About Healthy Living*. Ventura, CA: Regal, 1996.

Menopause

Budoff, Penny Wise. *No More Hot Flashes*. New York: Warner Books, 1984.

Greenwood, Sadja. *Menopause Naturally*. Volcano, CA: Volcano Press, 1992.

Ojeda, Linda. *Menopause Without Medicine*. Alameda, CA: Hunter House, 1992.

General Interest

Backus, William. *The Healing Power of a Christian Mind*. Minneapolis: Bethany House Publishers, 1996.

Borg, Marcus J. *Meeting Jesus for the First Time*. New York: Harper SanFrancisco, 1984.

Canfield, Jack et al. *Chicken Soup for the Christian Soul*. Deerfield Beach, FL: Health Communications, Inc., 1997.

Hager, W. David. *As Jesus Cared for Women*. Grand Rapids, MI: Revell, 1998.

Little, Paul. *Know Why You Believe*. Wheaton, IL: Victor Books, 1987.

McGinnis, Alan Loy, *The Balanced Life*. Minneapolis: Augsburg, 1997.

Palms, Roger. *Bible Readings on Hope*. Minneapolis: World Wide Publications, 1995.

Remus, Harold. *Jesus As Healer*. New York: Cambridge Press, 1997.

Siegel, Bernie. *Prescriptions for Living*. New York: Harper Collins, 1998.

More Sound Health Advice From J. Ron Eaker, MD

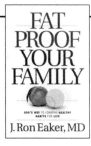

Healthy Living for the Whole Family!

Good nutrition and sound lifestyle choices can make your family trimmer, healthier, and happier—and *Fat-Proof Your Family* can show you how to get there.

Based on years of medical research and practice, Dr. Eaker gives you simple, straightforward tools to raise a healthy family, long term. Using biblical principles, Dr. Eaker helps you set goals beyond simple weight-loss management, showing how the whole family can achieve greater physical, spiritual and emotional health that will last a lifetime.

Fat-Proof Your Family by J. Ron Eaker, MD